# Fundamentals of Anaesthesia and Acute Medicine
# Local and Regional Anaesthesia

# FUNDAMENTALS OF ANAESTHESIA AND ACUTE MEDICINE

Series editors

**Ronald M Jones,** Professor of Anaesthetics, St Mary's Hospital Medical School, London, UK
**Alan R Aitkenhead,** Professor of Anaesthetics, University of Nottingham, UK
**Pierre Foëx,** Nuffield Professor of Anaesthetics, University of Oxford, UK

Titles already available:

*Anaesthesia for Obstetrics and Gynaecology*
Edited by Robin Russell

*Cardiovascular Physiology* (second edition)
Edited by Hans Joachim Priebe and Karl Skarvan

*Clinical Cardiovascular Medicine in Anaesthesia*
Edited by Pierre Coriat

*Intensive Care Medicine*
Edited by Julian Bion

*Management of Acute and Chronic Pain*
Edited by Narinder Rawal

*Neuro-Anaesthetic Practice*
Edited by H Van Aken

*Neuromuscular Transmission*
Edited by Leo HDJ Booij

*Paediatric Intensive Care*
Edited by Alan Duncan

Forthcoming:

*Day Care Anaesthesia*
Edited by Ian Smith

*Preoperative Assessment*
Edited by Jeremy Cashman

*Pharmacology of the Critically Ill*
Edited by Maire Shelly and Gilbert Park

Fundamentals of Anaesthesia and Acute Medicine

# Local and Regional Anaesthesia

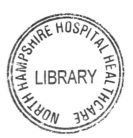

**Edited by**
Per H Rosenberg

*Professor of Anaesthesiology*
*Helsinki University*
*Finland*

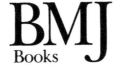

© BMJ Books 2000

BMJ Books is an imprint of the BMJ Publishing Group
www.bmjbooks.com

**British Library Cataloguing in Publication Data**
A catalogue record of this book is available
from the British Library

ISBN 0-7279-1480-4


Cover by Landmark Design, Croydon, Surrey
Typeset in Great Britain by
Phoenix Photosetting, Chatham, Kent
Printed and bound in Great Britain by
MPG Books Ltd, Bodmin, Cornwall

# Contents

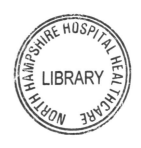

# Contributors

Jean-Jacques Eledjam
Department of Anaesthesia and Pain Clinic
University Hospital of Nimes and Medical School of Montpellier-Nimes,
France

Karl F Hampl
Department of Anaesthesia
University of Basel/Kantonsspital, Switzerland

Jan Jakobsson
Department of Anaesthsia
Sabbatsberg Hospital, Stockholm, Sweden

Michael Möllmann
Department of Anaesthesiology and Intensive Care
St Franziskus-Hospital, Münster, Germany

Steen Petersen-Felix
Institut für Anästhesiologie
University of Bern, Inselspital, Switzerland

Mikko T Pitkänen
Department of Anaesthesia
Helsinki University Central Hospital, Finland

Jacques Ripart
Department of Anaesthesia and Pain Clinic
University Hospital of Nimes and Medical School of Montpellier-Nimes,
France

Per H Rosenberg
Department of Anaesthesiology and Intensive Care Medicine
Helsinki University Central Hospital, Finland

CONTRIBUTORS

Markus C Schneider
Department of Anaesthesia
University of Basel/Kantonsspital, Switzerland

Bernadette Th Veering
Department of Anesthesiology
Leiden University Medical Center, The Netherlands

Marcel Vercauteren
Department of Anaesthesia
University Hospital Antwerp, Belgium

Eric Viel
Department of Anaesthesia and Pain Clinic
University Hospital of Nimes and Medical School of Montepellier-Nimes, France

# Foreword

## The Fundamentals of Anaesthesia and Acute Medicine series

The pace of change within the biological sciences continues to increase and nowhere is this more apparent than in the specialities of anaesthesia, acute medicine, and intensive care. Although many practitioners continue to rely on comprehensive but bulky texts for reference, the accelerating rate of biomedical advances makes this source of information increasingly likely to be dated, even if the latest edition is used. The series *Fundamentals of Anaesthesia and Acute Medicine* aims to bring to the reader up-to-date and authoritative reviews of the principal clinical topics which make up the specialities. Each volume will cover the fundamentals of the topic in a comprehensive manner but will also emphasise recent developments of controversial issues.

International differences in the practice of anaesthesia and intensive care are now much less than in the past and the editors of each volume have commissioned chapters from acknowledged authorities throughout the world to assemble contributions of the highest possible calibre. Three volumes will appear annually and, as the pace and extent of clinically significant advances vary among the individual topics, new editions will be commissioned to ensure that practitioners will be in a position to keep abreast of the important developments within the specialities.

Not only does the pace of advance in biomedical science serve to justify the appearance of an international series of this nature but the current awareness of the need for more formal continuing education also underlines the timeliness of its appearance. The editors would welcome feedback from readers about the series, which is aimed at both established practitioners and trainees preparing for degrees and diplomas in anaesthesia and intensive care.

RONALD M JONES
ALAN R AITKENHEAD
PIERRE FOËX

# Introduction

The chapters collected for this book present the most recent knowledge in the field. This series should be regarded as "current concepts" of the clinical use of local and regional anaesthesia rather than as a "textbook of local and regional anaesthesia". There are already several excellent textbooks with detailed descriptions of how to perform various nerve blocks and therefore another book of that kind is not required at the moment. Instead, this book focuses on some of the most recent applications of regional anaesthesia, for example in the chapter on obstetric analgesia by Dr Vercauteren and in the chapter by Dr Schneider and co-workers on current controversies associated with the use of some common techniques. On the other hand, the basis of safe practice, i.e. good knowledge of clinical pharmacology and toxicology of the local anaesthetics, as presented by Dr Veering and by Drs Rosenberg and Eledjam in their respective chapters, can never be emphasised too strongly. In today's practice, unfortunately, life-threatening toxicity complications still occur, almost always due to neglect of safety rules. The clinician must be able to recognise toxicity signs and symptoms at their initial appearance and must also be able to treat more severe toxic complications. Other complications which may occur in the practice of regional anaesthesia are explained by Dr Eledjam and his colleagues. Fortunately, such complications are rare but they can be avoided by good clinical judgement and meticulous technique.

Day surgery (outpatient surgery) is a growing field. Development of surgical techniques and anaesthetic agents, improvement in postoperative pain control, and sociomedical economic constraints have influenced this and one may predict that in the near future up to 60% of surgical operations will be performed on an outpatient basis. Local and regional anaesthesia may play an important role in reducing morbidity and expediting safe patient discharge, as described by Dr Jakobsson.

Some important practical principles of the most common local anaesthetic blocks, which can be used for both outpatient and inpatient surgical anaesthesia, are presented by Dr Rosenberg ("Common nerve blocks") and Dr Pitkänen ("Intravenous regional anaesthesia"). Dr Möllmann reviews the latest developments and experiences of needles, catheters, and other equipment used for regional anaesthesia.

Finally, it should be emphasised once more that this book, written by experts in the field of local and regional anaesthesia, must be regarded as a presentation of the "current status" of this constantly developing clinical field, as the applications for surgical anaesthesia as well as for analgesia in patients with acute or chronic pain will continue to expand.

I therefore recommend this book to anaesthesiologists as well as to other physicians who are involved in the clinical use of local anaesthetics and who wish to refresh their knowledge of the clinical practice of modern local and regional anaesthesia.

Per H Rosenberg

# 1: Clinical pharmacology of local anaesthetics

BERNADETTE Th VEERING

Although local anaesthetics have been used in clinical practice for more than a century, most of the current knowledge about their pharmacology has been derived from studies conducted during the last 20 years.

Electrophysiological studies have revealed much about their mechanisms of action, whereas determination of the blood and urine concentration profiles following various regional anaesthetic procedures has provided worthwhile information regarding their pharmacokinetics and fate in the body.

Understanding the pharmacology of local anaesthetics and their pharmacokinetic principles may help the clinician to select the most appropriate agent and dosage regimen for any particular application.

## Mechanism of action

### Sodium channels

Local anaesthetics block the generation and propogation of action potentials in excitable nerve tissues primarily by impairing the function of voltage-gated sodium ($Na^+$) channels in the axonal membrane.[1] The sodium channel itself is a specific receptor for local anaesthetic molecules.[2] Binding affinities of a local anaesthetic to the sodium channels are stereo selective; the (+)-enantiomers are more potent than (–)-enantiomers in inhibiting the normal $Na^+$ channel (Fig. 1.1).[3] Local anaesthetic agents inhibit the conformational changes that underlie channel activation and thereby prevent the opening of the channels.[1,2] As a consequence the sodium ion permeability of a stimulated membrane, and thereby the rate and degree of depolarisation, decrease progressively with increasing local anaesthetic concentrations. When depolarisation is insufficient to reach the threshold, full action potentials do not develop and conduction block occurs.

Local anaesthetics bind to a receptor in the channel that can be reached

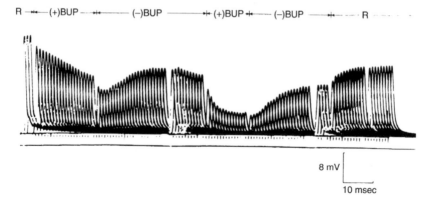

Fig 1.1   A series of compound action potentials in frog sciatic nerve, stimulated at 1/min, tracks the potency of bupivacaine (BUP) stereoisomers. The (+)-isomer of bupivacaine exhibits a greater tonic inhibitory potency compared to the (–)-isomer (reproduced with permission from Lee-Son et al[3])

by hydrophilic or hydrophobic pathways.[4] Both the charged and the neutral base forms of tertiary amine local anaesthetics are able to block sodium ion channels in excitable cell membranes. The charged form interacts from the cell interior via the hydrophilic pathway, whereas the neutral base form approaches the target structure from the lipophilic membrane phase, utilising the hydrophobic pathway.

### Frequency-dependent block

Local anaesthetic agents bind preferentially to open sodium channels and are released faster than they are bound by resting channels. Thus, the state of the channel (open, inactivated, closed or resting) affects the quality (depth) of block, i.e. so-called state-dependent block.[5] As the frequency of stimulation is increased, membrane ion channels are open and exposed to the drug more frequently. Consequently an additional increment of the degree of blockade (phasic or "frequency-dependent" inhibition) occurs. Thus a resting nerve is less sensitive to local anaesthetic-induced conduction blockade than a nerve that has been repetitively stimulated. The resting transmembrane potential or threshold potential is not altered by local anaesthetics. Association and dissociation of local anaesthetics with sodium channels are very fast processes and as such are not the major determinants of the time course of a nerve block.

In addition to $Na^+$ channels, local anaesthetics can also bind to other membrane-bound proteins. In particular, they can also block certain potassium channels.[6] The greater the inhibition of potassium channels, the more the potency is reduced.

## Minimum concentration

The minimum concentration necessary to produce conduction blockade of nerve impulses is termed $C_m$. It is the drug concentration that just halts impulse traffic, blocks the nerve and provides regional anaesthesia. The $C_m$ represents a dynamic equilibrium between channel-bound and channel-released drug, such that the net sodium current is decreased below the firing threshold level.[7] Each local anaesthetic agent has its own $C_m$, reflecting differing potencies of each drug.

Drug behaviour also depends on the environment, so $C_m$ must be further defined by the prevailing solution conditions, such as pH and temperature.[8,9] Dispersion, dilution by tissue fluid, destruction, tissue barriers, absorption by fat, uptake into the vasculature and local metabolism are all factors that determine the clinical potency. The final concentration of drug eventually arriving at the nerve depends on the relative magnitude of these factors and on the length of nerve exposed to drug solution.

## Differential blockade

Local anaesthetics are capable of blocking all kinds of nerve fibres. The different sensitivities of nerves to local anaesthetics result in clinically important zones of differential blockade involving somatic motor fibres, somatic sensory fibres and preganglionic sympathetic fibres. This phenomenon of selective blockade was considered to depend upon differences in diffusion of local anaesthetics into fibres, related to their $pK_a$ and lipid solubility. In addition, it has been postulated that differences in the minimum concentration necessary to block axons of different diameters, fibre size, myelinisation and frequency of incoming impulses contribute to differential blockade.[10,11] More recently, it has been emphasised that the susceptibility to conduction block is not correlated to fibre size per se but to the length of exposed segment and the number of nodes it contains.[12,13] A possible explanation for this sensorimotor dissociation is that the length of nerve in the dural root sleeves exposed to local anaesthetic is not sufficient to allow block of three consecutive nodes of Ranvier in the myelinated A-α motor fibres, because of the large internodal distances, but is sufficient to block unmyelinated C pain fibres and produce a three-node block in myelinated A-δ pain fibres, which have smaller internodal distances.

## Structure

Local anaesthetics are organic amines, with an intermediary ester or amide linkage separating the lipophilic ring-linked head from the hydrophilic hydrocarbon tail (Fig. 1.2).[14] The nature of this bond is the basis for classifying the drugs as ester local anaesthetics or amide local anaesthetics. The hydrophilic group is generally a secondary or tertiary amine, while the lipophilic group is usually an aromatic residue. The amino amides include lignocaine, mepivacaine, prilocaine, ropivacaine, bupivacaine and etidocaine. The amino esters include procaine, chloroprocaine and amethocaine (tetracaine).

The chemical difference is reflected biologically in the site of metabolism: ester-type agents are mainly hydrolysed by pseudocholinesterases in plasma and elsewhere while amide compounds undergo enzymatic degradation predominantly in the liver. The chemical difference is also revealed in the allergic potential: a higher frequency of allergic reactions is observed with the ester-type agents that are derivates of *p*-aminobenzoic acid.

## Physicochemical properties and local anaesthetic action

The various local anaesthetic agents differ in terms of their potency, onset, and duration of action. These clinical properties are partly dependent

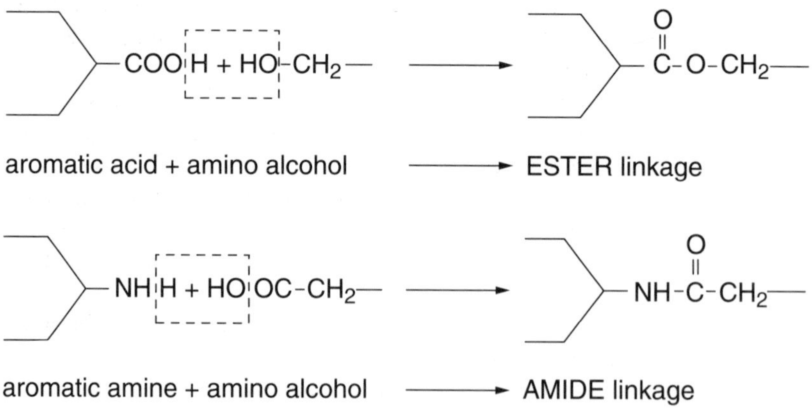

Fig 1.2  Ester or amide linkages are forged when aromatic and amino fractions combine; one molecule of water (dashed boxes) splits off (reproduced with permission from de Jong RH, ed. *Local anesthetics*. St Louis: Mosby, 1994: 101)

on their physicochemical properties, such as dissociation constant ($pK_a$), lipid solubility, and protein binding. These relationships are essentially what is observed in in vitro nerve models but in vivo, other actions of the local anaesthetics, such as vasodilator properties, may also influence the anaesthetic profile.

Structural alterations in the molecule produce physicochemical changes that can alter anaesthetic potency. The lipid solubility is an important determinant of anaesthetic potency, normally expressed in terms of partition coefficient. This is the ratio of concentration that the drug develops when it is dissolved in a mixture of a lipid and an aqueous solvent.[15] Changes in either the aromatic or amine portion of a local anaesthetic can alter lipid solubility and thereby affect anaesthetic potency.

An increase in degree of protein binding is thought to increase the duration of local anaesthetic activity. Proteins account for approximately 10% of the nerve membrane. Therefore, agents that penetrate the axolemma and attach more firmly to membrane proteins have a prolonged duration of anaesthetic activity. The dissociation constant ($pK_a$) of a chemical compound is the pH at which the concentration of ionised and non-ionised forms is equal. Local anaesthetics are weak bases with $pK_a$ values that range from 7.6 to 8.9 (Table 1.1). Since it is the uncharged base that diffuses across the nerve sheath, the onset of anaesthesia is related to the amount of drug in the base form.

The percentage of local anaesthetic in the base form, when injected into tissue whose pH is 7.4, is inversely proportional to the $pK_a$ of that agent. Local anaesthetics with a $pK_a$ near physiological pH (7.4) have a greater amount of drug in the non-ionised form (which more readily diffuses across the nerve sheath and membrane to its site of action) than local anaesthetics with a higher $pK_a$. Studies on isolated nerves confirm that local anaesthetics like lignocaine, whose pH is closer to tissue pH, have a more rapid onset than agents with a high $pK_a$, such as amethocaine.[16]

The onset of action in vivo may be altered by the rate of diffusion through non-nervous tissue and the concentration of local anaesthetic employed for various regional anaesthetic procedures. For example, 0.25% bupivacaine possesses a rather slow onset of action. However, increasing the concentration of bupivacaine to 0.75% results in a significant decrease in the onset of action. This may be related to the larger number of molecules placed in the vicinity of nerves.

The effect of local anaesthetic agents on the vasculature at the site of injection also influences the in vivo potency and duration of action of these compounds. For example, lignocaine causes a greater degree of vasodilatation than either mepivacaine or prilocaine, resulting in a more rapid vascular absorption of lignocaine such that fewer molecules of lignocaine are available to block nerves in vivo.[17] Local anaesthetics exhibit a direct biphasic action on vascular smooth muscle, depending upon the local

*Table 1.1 Physicochemical properties of local anaesthetics (reproduced with permission from Cousins MJ, Bridenbaugh PO. Neural blockade. In: Clinical anesthesia and management of pain, 3rd edn. Philadelphia: Lippincott, 1998: 56.*

| | Chemical configuration | | | Physiochemical properties | | | |
|---|---|---|---|---|---|---|---|
| Agent | Aromatic lipophilic | Intermediate chain | Amine hydrophilic | Molecular weight (Base) | pK$_a$ (25°C) | Partitition coefficient | Percent protein binding |
| *Esters* | | | | | | | |
| Benzocaine | H$_2$N— | —COOCH$_2$CH$_3$ | | 165 | 2.5 | 81 | ? |
| Butamben | H$_2$N— | —COO(CH$_2$)$_3$ CH$_3$ | | 193 | 2.3 | 1028 | ? |
| Procaine | H$_2$N— | —COOCH$_2$CH$_2$—N | C$_2$H$_5$ / C$_2$H$_5$ | 236 | 9.05 | 1.7 | 6 |
| Chloroprocaine | H$_2$N— (Cl) | —COOCH$_2$CH$_2$—N | C$_2$H$_5$ / C$_2$H$_5$ | 271 | 8.97 | 9.0 | ? |
| Amethocaine | H$_9$C$_4$N—H | —COOCH$_2$CH$_2$—N | CH$_3$ / CH$_3$ | 264 | 8.46 | 221 | 75.6 |
| *Amides* | | | | | | | |
| Prilocaine | CH$_3$ | NHCOCH—CH$_3$ | —N—H / C$_3$H$_7$ | 220 | 7.9 | 25 | 55 approx. |
| Lignocaine | | NHCOCH$_2$— | N—C$_2$H / C$_2$H$_5$ | 234 | 7.91 | 2.4 | 64 |
| Etidocaine | | NHCOCH$_2$—C$_2$H$_5$ | N—C$_2$H$_5$ / C$_3$H$_7$ | 276 | 7.7 | 800 | 94 |
| Mepivacaine | CH$_3$ / CH$_3$ | NHCO— | N—CH$_3$ | 246 | 7.76 | 21 | 77 |
| Ropivacaine | | NHCO— | N—C$_3$H$_7$ | 262 | 8.2 | 115 | 95 |
| Bupivacaine | | NHCO— | N—C$_4$H$_9$ | 288 | 8.16 | 346 | 96 |

anaesthetic agent, its concentration and stereochemical configuration, the type of blood vessel (capacitance or resistance) and preexisting vascular tone.[18] At low concentrations local anaesthetics cause vasoconstriction. At concentrations used for epidural anaesthesia, they tend to be vasodilators (except for ropivacaine).

## Classification

Based on differences in anaesthetic potency and duration of action in man, it is possible to divide local anaesthetic agents into three categories.

(1) Agents of low anaesthetic potency and short duration of action: procaine and chloroprocaine.
(2) Agents of intermediate anaesthetic potency and duration of action: lignocaine, mepivacaine and prilocaine.
(3) Agents of high anaesthetic potency and prolonged duration of action: amethocaine, ropivacaine, bupivacaine, and etidocaine.

## Stereoisomers

With the exception of lignocaine, most of the commercially available local anaesthetic drugs are racemic mixtures containing a chiral centre and consequently exist in two optically active, stereoisomeric forms (enantiomers). Enantiomers can and frequently do have different pharmacological and pharmacokinetic properties.[19] Clinically, local anaesthetic agents are used as racemic mixtures containing equal amounts of both enantiomers.

Racemic bupivacaine has a chiral centre and exists as two enantiomers: levobupivacaine (also known as L- or S-bupivacaine) and dexbupivacaine (also known as D- or R-bupivacaine) in a 50:50 ratio (Fig. 1.3). The enantiomers of bupivacaine have identical physicochemical properties but their pharmacologic and toxicologic effects differ because of stereoselective differences in binding of the drug to relevant receptors for drug activity, distribution, and metabolism.[20] Animal experiments have shown greater toxicity of the R(+) enantiomer compared with the S(−)enantiomer.[21] S(−)-bupivacaine is less toxic to the CNS than R(+)-bupivacaine and produces fewer cardiac conduction disturbances than either rac-bupivacaine or R(+)-bupivacaine.[22] Based on these data, S(−)-bupivacaine will probably have a greater margin of safety than racemic bupivacaine and is being extensively investigaged in the clinical setting.

In contrast to mepivacaine and bupivacaine, ropivacaine has been developed as a pure S-enantiomer.[23]

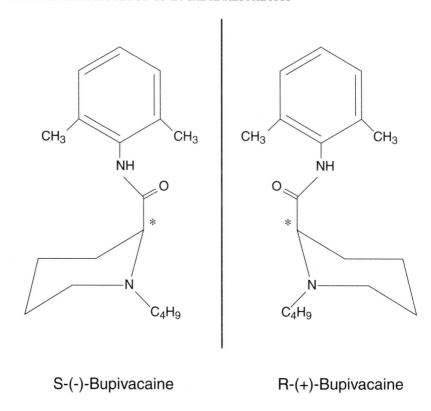

S-(-)-Bupivacaine                R-(+)-Bupivacaine

Fig 1.3   Enantiomers of bupivacaine

## Individual drug properties

The local anaesthetics available for clinical use are summarised in Table 1.1.

### Esters

*Cocaine*

Cocaine is an ester of benzoic acid. It provides excellent topical anaesthesia and is the only local anaesthetic that produces vasoconstriction at clinically useful concentrations. For this reason it is commonly used to shrink swollen mucosal membrane in daily clinical otorhinolaryngologic practice in concentrations of 4–10%. Because of its addictive properties, associated with a relatively high potential for systemic toxicity and tendency to produce allergic reactions, cocaine is only used for topical anaesthesia.

*Procaine*

Procaine is a derivative of *p*-aminobenzoic acid. It is rarely used because of its low potency, slow onset, and relatively short duration of action. It is currently used mainly for infiltration anaesthesia in concentrations of 0.5%. Some centres use procaine 5–10% for short-acting spinal anaesthesia and for differential spinal anaesthesia at concentrations of 5% in chronic pain patients. Procaine is hydrolysed to *p*-aminobenzoic acid, which may cause allergic-type reactions. Rapid hydrolysis of procaine accounts for its low systemic toxicity.

*Chloroprocaine*

Chloroprocaine differs from procaine by the addition of a chlorine atom to the aromatic ring. It has a rapid onset and a short duration of action. It is hydrolysed some four times faster than procaine in human plasma, resulting in low toxicity and a short duration of action. It is primarily used for epidural analgesia in obstetrics.

*Amethocaine*

Amethocaine, called tetracaine in the United States, is the butylaminobenzoic acid derivative of procaine. It is a potent, long-acting local anaesthetic that produces a high degree of motor block, with excellent qualities of sensory block. It is used primarily for spinal anaesthesia in hypobaric, hyperbaric or isobaric solution. Amethocaine is used for topical anaesthesia of the eye but rarely for other forms of regional anaesthesia because of its extremely slow onset of action and the potential for systemic toxic reactions when the larger doses required for other types of regional blockade are used.

*Butamben*

Butyl aminobenzoate (BAB) is an amino ester local anaesthetic with extraordinary physiochemical characteristics: a very low $pK_a$, a very high partition coefficient, and an extremely low water solubility (Table 1.1). When given as a suspension, epidural administration of BAB to cancer patients caused ultra-long lasting analgesia up to six months, without motor block.[24] Thus, the promising pharmacodynamic properties of BAB in a small number of cancer patients clearly warrant further evaluation of the efficacy and safety of the BAB suspension.

## Amides

*Lignocaine*

Lignocaine is the most versatile and commonly used local anaesthetic agent as a result of its rapid onset of action, inherent potency, and moderate duration of action. It is used in concentrations of 0.5% to 5%, depending on the mode of application. It is the agent of choice for short procedures but to prolong its duration of action of lignocaine and enhance its systemic safety, a vasoconstrictor (commonly adrenaline) is frequently added.

## Prilocaine

Prilocaine is an aminoamide local anaesthetic derived from a toluidine derivative and a tertiary amine. It has a clinical profile similar to that of lignocaine, i.e., a relatively rapid onset of action while providing a moderate duration of anaesthesia and a profound depth of neural blockade. A disadvantage of prilocaine is that higher doses result in methaemoglobinaemia.[25] Because of this, its use is limited to single injection procedures.

Prilocaine is used in concentrations of 0.5% to 2%, depending on the mode of application.

## Mepivacaine

Mepivacaine is structurally related to lignocaine. Its duration of action is somewhat longer than that of lignocaine when each agent is used without adrenaline. It has less vasodilatory action but it is also less versatile. The addition of adrenaline prolongs the duration of action of mepivacaine by approximately 75%. It is used in concentrations of 0.5% to 2%, depending on the mode of application.

## Bupivacaine

Bupivacaine belongs to the long-acting aminoamide class of local anaesthetics. It is a homologue of mepivacaine but possesses a greater anaesthetic potency and more prolonged duration of action. It is a weak base and has a $pK_a$ of 8.1. Other physicochemical properties of bupivacaine are summarised in Table 1.1

Bupivacaine has the ability to provide differential blocks of sensory and motor fibres, particularly at low concentrations. As a result, it is used successfully for obstetric anaesthesia and postoperative pain management, for which analgesia without significant motor block is highly desirable. It is administered in concentrations of 0.06% to 0.75%, depending on the mode of administration.

## Etidocaine

Etidocaine is structurally similar to lignocaine. It has a great lipid solubility and near-total plasma protein binding. This agent is characterised by very rapid onset, prolonged duration of action, and profound motor blockade. Because of this, it is used mainly for surgical procedures in which profound motor block is required. It is administered in concentrations of 1% to 1.5%.

*Ropivacaine*

Ropivacaine is the first enantiomerically pure local anaesthetic and exists as the S-enantiomer. It is chemically homologous to bupivacaine and mepivacaine and has an intermediate lipid solubility approximately one-third that of racemic bupivacaine. Plasma protein binding and $pK_a$ value are similar to those of bupivacaine (see Table 1.1). It was developed in response to reports of cardiac toxicity associated mainly with epidural administration of 0.75% bupivacaine. The well-publicised rationale for ropivacaine is for long duration of neural blockade with a lower risk of cardiovascular toxicity and an even greater sensorimotor dissociation (differential blockade) than with bupivacaine.[23]

## Miscellaneous

*Articaine*

Articaine belongs to the anilide group of local anaesthetics, similar to lignocaine and mepivacaine, although it differs from these agents in that it has a toluidine ring instead of a benzene ring in its stucture. It is a thiophene derivative (containing a sulphur atom in its molecule) and is commonly used in dentistry in some countries.

*Dibucaine*

Dibucaine is a quinoline derivative with an amide bond in the intermediate chain. It is very toxic and this limits its use to spinal anaesthesia.

# Eutectic mixture of local anaesthetics (EMLA)

EMLA is a eutectic mixture of the base forms of lignocaine and prilocaine, in an oil-in-water emulsion containing approximately 80% active local anaesthetic.[26] This mixture produces effective topical analgesia in normal skin within 0.5–1 hour. After diffusion to deeper skin layers, selective uptake in nervous tissues contributes to the analgesia. EMLA is especially useful in children before venous puncture and for dermatological surgery.[27] Plasma levels of both anaesthetics following application are far below toxic levels both in infants (3–12 months) and adults.[28] Nevertheless, EMLA cream has to be handled with caution since there is only limited experience regarding cutaneous resorption and toxic limits in children.

# Liposomal local anaesthetics

Liposomes are microscopic spheres that consist of a phospholipid bilayer that encapsulates an aqueous core. They have been found to enhance the therapeutic properties of local anaesthetics. The local anaesthetic is released slowly from the liposome depot and thus the duration of action of the nerve blockade will be prolonged.[29] In particular, administration of lignocaine or bupivacaine in liposomes has been shown to prolong the duration of epidural anaesthesia.[30]

## Factors influencing anaesthetic activity

### Dosage of local anaesthetic

The total dose (i.e. product of volume and concentration) is probably the main determinant of the pharmocodynamic profile of a local anaesthetic agent. An increase in the dose of local anaesthetic produces a faster onset and a longer duration of sensory block and increasing the concentration results in a faster onset and a more profound motor block.

The dose of local anaesthetic administered must be tailored to where the drug is injected, because the toxic effects of a local anaesthetic depend on the rapidity of absorption from an injection site and the total dose injected. Regardless of the local anaesthetic used, the rate of absorption usually decreases in the following sequence: interpleural, intercostal, caudal, epidural, brachial plexus, subcutaneous, sciatic and femoral block (Fig. 1.4).[31] Adding adrenaline decreases the peak plasma concentrations of local anaesthetic agents but the degree of this reduction depends on the site of injection and the specific local anaesthetic agent.[31] A recommended maximum dose should be related to the site of injection in addition to the presence or absence of adrenaline (see Table 2.1, pp. 23–24).

### Addition of a vasoconstrictor

The quality of a regional block may be improved by the concomitant use of a vasoconstrictor, particularly adrenaline. This effect may be related to a decrease in blood flow at the site of injection, leading to decreased vascular absorption and increased neuronal uptake of local anaesthetic.[31] As a consequence the depth and duration of neural blockade are increased.

The effects of adrenaline on the quality of a regional block vary markedly with the site of injection and the type, dose, and concentration of the local anaesthetic. For example, the addition of adrenaline to all local anaesthetic solutions significantly prolongs the duration of action of infiltration anaesthesia and peripheral nerve blocks but the addition of adrenaline to prilocaine, etidocaine, and bupivacaine has little or no effect on the duration of action of epidural anaesthesia.[32] However, the addition of adrenaline to lignocaine and mepivacaine markedly prolongs the duration of action of epidural anaesthesia.[33] This differential effect may be related to the

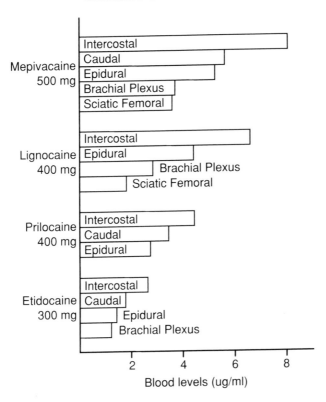

Fig 1.4  Comparative peak venous blood concentrations of several local anaesthetic agents after administration into various anatomic sites (reproduced with permission from Covino BG, Vassallo HG. *Local anesthetics: mechanisms of action and clinical use.* New York: Grune and Stratton, 1976: 97)

differences in physicochemical properties (for example, local binding) and the intrinsic vasoactivity of the agents. The effects of adding adrenaline are more important when the concentration of the local anaesthetic solution is low than when it is high. The optimal concentration of adrenaline is 1:200 000 (5 µg/ml), although lower concentrations are sometimes recommended in obstetrics.

## Pharmacokinetics

The pharmacokinetics of local anaesthetics during a regional anaesthetic procedure consist of a local disposition, which is a process in which the drug distributes into and out of the tissues near the site of injection, a systemic absorption, and a systemic disposition (Fig. 1.5).[31] Local distribution involves several processes, including spread of the local anaesthetic by bulk flow, diffusion, transport via blood vessels, and binding to local tissues. Local disposition determines the time course of the concentration of local anaesthetic at the sites of action. The local disposition is difficult to assess because it requires measurements of concentrations in tissues and fluids. Consequently, investigations of the pharmacokinetics of local anaesthetic agents are focused on the systemic absorption and systemic disposition.

## Systemic absorption

Systemic absorption of local anaesthetics is of concern as a major determinant of the blood concentrations and the possible consequences in terms of systemic side effects and toxicity. Furthermore, knowledge of the absorption rate is important in relation to the clinical profile, in particular the duration of blockade. Systemic absorption is dependent on the binding of local anaesthetics to tissues at and near the site of injection, and on local perfusion.[31,34] Both vary with the site of injection. Furthermore, local anaesthetics may alter local perfusion, both by affecting vasomotor tone and by producing sympathetic block. Following a regional procedure injection, vasoactive properties of local anaesthetic agents may influence their own

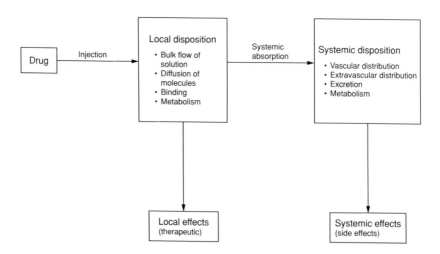

Fig 1.5   Fate of local anaesthetic agents (reproduced with permission from Mather LE, Cousins MJ. Local anaesthetics and their current clinical use. *Drugs* 1979; **18:** 185–205)

systemic absorption, by modifying local perfusion. The degree of vaso-activity is most prominent with the lipophilic long-acting agents such as bupivacaine and etidocaine, which is seldom used nowadays. However, their absorption rate is comparatively less than the absorption rate of ligno-caine and mepivacaine, probably because of greater tissue binding at the site of injection.[31]

All amide-type agents exhibit a biphasic pattern of systemic absorption, with an initial rapid phase followed by a much slower phase.[31,35,36] The rapid absorption phase is related to the initial high concentration gradient between the drug in the injected solution and the blood. The slow phase probably reflects absorption after local distribution has been completed. For example, the slower second absorption phase following epidural admin-istration of a local anaesthetic is believed to occur because of slow uptake of local anaesthetics sequestered in the epidural fat and will therefore depend upon tissue/blood partitioning. The slower absorption of bupivacaine compared to lignocaine probably reflects greater tissue affinity and is consistent with its longer duration of action.[37]

## Systemic disposition

### Lung uptake

The lung, through which all the absorbed drug passes before entering the arterial blood, appears to be important in the initial distribution of amide-type local anaesthetics in the body.[38] Studies with lignocaine have demonstrated a first-pass uptake of approximately 60%. However, the initial high uptake is followed by quite a rapid release. Therefore, the lung may be considered as a buffer which dampens the rapid increase of the arterial concentration of local anaesthetics in cases of accidental intravenous injection, such as accidental premature cuff release during intravenous regional anaesthesia. The tissue uptake is dependent on tissue blood flow, lipid content, pH gradient, membrane permeability, and plasma drug binding.[39]

Differences in lung uptake may exist between the various local anaes-thetic agents based on differences in their physiochemical properties. In addition, lung uptake is reduced as the dose of local anaesthetics adminis-tered is increased. Lung uptake is promoted by the relatively low pH of lung water compared with plasma.

### Placental transfer

Equilibration between local anaesthetics in the umbilical vein and those in maternal blood occurs very rapidly, possibly within one circulation time.[40] Total umbilical venous/maternal venous plasma concentrations ratios may be considerably less than unity. This low ratio reflects different maternal and foetal plasma binding of local anaesthetics owing to considerably lower concentrations of $\alpha_1$-acid glycoprotein in the foetal plasma than in the maternal plasma.[31] Unbound concentrations (free active drug concentrations) are likely to be similar in foetal and maternal blood.[31] Local anaesthetics are weak bases and their placental transfer is enhanced by foetal hypoxia and acidosis. The unbound concentrations are possibly somewhat higher in the acidotic foetus due to ion trapping.[41]

Ester local anaesthetics, because of their rapid hydrolysis, are not available to cross the placenta in significant amounts.[42]

## Distribution

After systemic absorption local anaesthetics are rapidly distributed to the highly perfused organs (kidney, lung, etc.) and more slowly to less perfused tissues such as skeletal muscle and fat.

As they are lipophilic compounds, the tissue distribution of local anaesthetics will be highly dependent upon tissue perfusion (vascularity). Local anaesthetic agents in the blood are predominantly bound to $\alpha_1$-acid glycoprotein (AAG), a high-affinity, low-capacity protein, and to a lesser degree to albumin, which is a low-affinity, high-capacity protein.[43] The more potent and longer acting local anaesthetics are bound more extensively to plasma and tissue protein. Extensive tissue uptake of local anaesthetics limits the significance of plasma binding as a determinant of their overall distribution; a small percentage will remain in the blood at any time.[31]

Plasma protein binding of local anaesthetics should be taken into account when interpreting plasma concentrations of individual agents in relation to toxicity, since toxic effects are likely to be more closely related to free (unbound) plasma concentrations than to total blood or plasma concentrations.[44]

The distribution of local anaesthetics is to some extent enantioselective. The volume of distribution of R(–)-mepivacaine is approximately twice that of S(+)-mepivacaine and the volume of distribution of R(+)-bupivacaine is 50% larger than that of S(–)-bupivacaine.[45,46] The enantioselective systemic disposition of both local anaesthetics can to a large extent be attributed to  differences in the degree of plasma binding of the enantiomers.

## Elimination

Local anaesthetics are predominantly eliminated by metabolism. The amino amides are almost completely metabolised by enzymatic degradation, primarily in the liver, although prilocaine also undergoes substantial metabolism elsewhere in the body since the estimated total body clearance considerably exceeds liver blood flow. The amino esters are predominantly hydrolysed in blood by plasma pseudocholinesterases and red cell esterases at an extremely rapid rate.[47] The amino amides are almost completely metabolised by enzymatic degradation, primarily in the liver.[48] Just a very small amount of the parent drug is excreted unchanged via the kidney into the urine. This amount varies from up to 3% for lignocaine to less than 1% for bupivacaine.

Most studies concerning metabolism have been performed with lignocaine. Lignocaine biotransformation results in at least one active metabolite: monoethylglycinexylidide (MGEX) which is subsequently hydrolysed to xylidine.[49] Prilocaine biotransformation results in o-toluidine and subsequent formation of an N-hydroxy metabolite.[24] The latter may cause methaemoglobinaemia if the dose of prilocaine exceeds 600 mg in adults.

The clearance of mepivacaine[45] and bupivacaine[46] has been found to be stereoselective. The total plasma clearance of R(−)-mepivacaine was found to be significantly greater than that of S(+)-mepivacaine. From a toxicological point of view it is interesting to note that while the R(+) enantiomer of bupivacaine is cleared from plasma 1.25 times more rapidly than the S(−) form, the clearance based on unbound bupivacaine was 0.84 times lower.[46]

# Pharmacokinetic alterations by patient status and other drugs

Changes in body composition, hepatic blood flow, and hepatic mass that occur with normal ageing may have an impact on the rate and extent of the systemic absorption, distribution, metabolism, and excretion of local anaesthetics.[50] The clearance of lignocaine and bupivacaine decreases with age after epidural administration.[51,52] Plasma concentrations will probably rise to higher levels in older patients, which reduces the safety margin. Consequently infusion rates or top-up doses may need to be adjusted in older patients. The observed age-related decline in clearance of bupivacaine cannot be explained on the basis of changes in serum protein binding but probably reflects a concomitant decline in hepatic enzyme activity.[53]

Concomitant congestive heart failure, hypovolaemia, large blood loss, and hepatic diseases may alter the elimination of amino amides.[31]

Co-administered drugs like propranolol, cimetidine, and itraconazole have been shown to decrease the clearance of intravenously administered lignocaine and bupivacaine, mainly by direct inhibition of mixed function oxides activity, with a small contribution from decreased liver blood flow.[54–56]

17

The effect of multiple doses of cimetidine and ranitidine on bupivacaine clearance has not been determined.

# Conclusion

Local anaesthetic agents are drugs anaesthetists encounter every day. These agents provide a safe and efficacious method of preventing or relieving pain in circumscribed areas of the body. Local anaesthetic agents are effective drugs with known predictable toxicity when used properly.

The essential anaesthetic properties of these compounds are onset, potency, duration of action, and blockade of sensory and motor fibres. The pharmacologic activity of local anaesthetic agents is related primarily to their physiochemical properties. However, the activity of these agents in vivo may be altered by other actions, such as vasoactive properties which are essentially unrelated to the physiochemical properties of the various agents.

Most of the commercially available local anaesthetic drugs are racemic mixtures of their R and S enantiomers. However, there is evidence that the use of single S-enantiomer compounds offers advantages over racemic agents. This has led to the commercial production of ropivacaine, the enantiomerically [(S(–)] pure propyl homologue of bupivacaine. More recently, the S(–)-enantiomer of bupivacaine (already registered as levobupivacaine) has been extensively investigated in the clinical setting.

In considering the pharmacokinetics of local anaesthetics, both the systemic absorption and systemic disposition are of importance. Systemic absorption of local anaesthetics limits the duration of nerve block and is of concern in systemic toxicity. Reduction of the total plasma clearance of bupivacaine and lignocaine by increasing age and co-administered drugs like propranolol and cimetidine may result in significant accumulation of plasma concentrations following long-term continuous epidural infusions. Infusion rates or top-up doses may need to be adjusted. Further investigation is needed to determine effective minimal dose requirements in this group of patients.

Prudent use of local anaesthetics requires knowledge of their pharmacokinetics, pharmacodynamics and toxicity, technical skill in the performance of regional anaesthetic procedures, an evaluation of the patient's clinical status, and estimation of surgical requirements and duration of postoperative analgesia.

1  Butterworth JF IV, Strichartz GR. Molecular mechanism of local anesthesia: a review. *Anesthesiology* 1990:72:711–34.
2  Strichartz GR. The inhibition of sodium currents in myelinated nerve by quarternary derivatives of lidocaine. *J Gen Physiol* 1973;**62**:37–57.

3   Lee-Son S, Wang GK, Concus A, Crill E, Strichartz G. Stereo selective inhibition of neuronal sodium channels by local anesthetics. *Anesthesiology* 1992;**77**:324–35.

4   Hille B. Local anesthetics: hydrophilic and hydrophobic pathways for the drug-receptor reactions. *J Gen Physiol* 1977;**69**:497–515.

5   Courtney KR, Kendig JJ, Cohen EN. The rates of interaction of local anesthetics with sodium channels in nerve. *J Pharmacol Exp Ther* 1978;**207**:594–604.

6   Courtney KR, Kendig JJ. Bupivacaine is an effective potassium channel blocker in the heart. *Biochim Biophys Acta* 1988;**939**:163–6.

7   Fink BR, Cairns AM. Lack of size-related differential sensitivity to equilibrium conduction block among mammalian myelinated axons exposed to lidocaine. *Anesth Analg* 1987;**66**:948–53.

8   Wong K, Strichartz GR, Raymond SA. On the mechanism of potentiation of local anesthetics by bicarbonate buffer: drug structure-activity studied on isolated peripheral nerve. *Anesth Analg* 1993;**76**:131–43.

9   Rosenberg PH, Heavner JE. Temperature-dependent nerve-blocking action of lidocaine and halothane. *Acta Anaesth Scand* 1980;**24**:314–43.

10  Gissen AJ, Covino BG, Gregus J. Differential sensitivities of mammalian nerve fibres to local anesthetic agents. *Anesthesiology* 1980:**53**:467–74.

11  Wildsmith JAW, Brown DT, Paul D, Johnson S. Structure-activity relationships in differential nerve block at high and low frequency stimulation. *Br J Anaesth* 1989;**63**:444–52.

12  Fink BR. Mechnisms of differential axial blockade in epidural and subarachnoid anesthesia. *Anesthesiology* 1989;**70**:851–8.

13  Raymond SA, Steffensen SC, Gugino LD, Strichartz GR. The role of length of nerve exposed to local anesthetics in impulse blocking action. *Anesth Analg* 1989;**68**:563–70.

14  De Jong RH. *Local anesthetics*. St Louis: Mosby, 1994:101.

15  Sanchez V, Ferrante FM, Cibotti N, Strichartz GR. Partitioning of tetracaine base and cation into phospholipid membranes: relevance to anesthetic potency (abstract). *Reg Anesth* 1988;**13**(Suppl):81.

16  Ritchie JM, Ritchie BR. Local anesthetics: effects of pH on activity. *Science* 1968;**162**:1394–5.

17  Johns RA, DiFazio CA, Longnecker DE. Lidocaine constricts or dilates rat arterioles in a dose-dependent manner. *Anesthesiology* 1985;**62**:141–4.

18  Löfström JB. Ulnar nerve blockade for the evaluation for the anaesthetic agents. *Br J Anaesth* 1975;**47**:297–333.

19  Tucker GT, Lennard MS. Enantiomer specific pharmacokinetics. *Pharmacol Ther* 1990;**45**:309–29.

20  Gristwood R, Bardsley H, Baker H, Dickens J. Reduced cardiotoxicity of levobupivacaine compared with racemic bupivacaine (Marcaine): new clinical evidence. *Exp Opin Invest Drug* 1994;**3**:1209–12.

21  Huang YF, Pryor ME, Mather LE, Veering BT. Cardiovascular and central nervous system effects of intravenous levobupivacaine and bupivacaine in sheep. *Anesth Analg* 1998;**86**:797–804.

22  Bardsley H, Gristwood R, Baker H, Watson N, Nimmo W. A comparison of the cardiovascular effects of levobupivacaine and rac-bupivacaine following intravenous administration to healthy volunteers. *Br J Clin Pharmacol* 1998:**46**:245–9.

23 Markham A, Faulds D. Ropivacaine: a review of its pharmacology and thera-peutic use in regional anaesthesia. *Drugs* 1996;**52**:429–49.

24 Korsten HHM, Ackerman EW, Grouls RJE *et al.* Long-lasting epidural sensory blockade by n-butyl-p-aminobenzoate in the terminally ill intractable cancer patient. *Anesthesiology* 1991;**75**:950–60.

25 Hjelm M, Holmdahl MH. Biochemical effects of aromatic amines. II. Cyanosis, methaemoglobinaemia and Heinz-body formation induced by a local anaes-thetic agent (prilocaine). *Acta Anaesthesiol Scand* 1965;**9**:99–120.

26 Brodin A, Nyqvist-Mayer A, Wadsten T, Forslund B, Broberg F. Phase diagram and aqueous solubility of the lidocaine-prilocaine binary system. J Pharm Sci 1984;**73**:481–4.

27 Buckley MM, Benfield P. Eutectic lidocaine/prilocaine cream. A review of the topical anaesthetic/analgesic efficacy of a eutectic mixture of local anaesthetics (EMLA). *Drugs* 1993;**46**:126–51.

28 Engberg G, Danielson K, Henneberg S, Nilsson A. Plasma concentrations of prilocaine and lidocaine and methaemoglobin formation in infants after epicu-taneous application of a 5% lidocaine-prilocaine cream (EMLA). *Acta Anaesthesiol Scand* 1987;**31**:624–8.

29 Boogaerts JG, Lafont ND, Declerq AG *et al.* Epidural administration of lipo-some associated bupivacaine for the management of postsurgical pain: a first study. *J Clin Anesth* 1994;**6**:315–20.

30 Duncan L, Wildsmith JAW. Liposomal local anaesthetics. *Br J Anaesth* 1995;**75**:260–1.

31 Tucker GT. Pharmacokinetics of local anaesthetic agents, *Br J Anaesth* 1986;**58**:717–31.

32 Sinclair CJ, Scott DB. Comparison of bupivacaine and etidocaine in extradural blockade. *Br J Anaesth* 1976;**56**:147–53.

33 Murphy TM, Mather LE, Stanton-Hicks MD, Bonica JJ, Tucker GT. The effects of adding adrenaline to etidocaine and lignocaine in extradural anaes-thesia. I: Block characteristics and cardiovascular effects. *Br J Anaesth* 1976;**48**:893–97.

34 Burm AGL. Clinical pharmacokinetics of epidural and spinal anaesthesia. *Clin Pharmacokinet* 1989;**16**:283–311.

35 Veering BT, Brum AGL, Vletter AA, van den Heuvel RPM, Onkenhout W, Spierdijk J. The effect of age on the systemic absorption and disposition of bupi-vacaine after epidural administration. *Clin Pharmacokinet* 1992;**22**:75–84.

36 Emanuelsson BM, Persson J, Alm C, Heller A, Gustafsson LL. Systemic absorption and block after epidural injection of ropivacaine in healthy volun-teers. *Anesthesiology* 1997;**87**:1309–17.

37 Burm AGL, Vermeulen NPE, van Kleef JW, de Boer AG, Spierdijk J, Breimer DD. Pharmacokinetics of lidocaine and bupivacaine in surgical patients fol-lowing epidural administration. Simultaneous investigation of absorption and disposition kinetics using stable isotopes. *Clin Pharmacokinet* 1987;**13**:191–203.

38 Jorfeldt L, Lewis DH, Löfström JB, Post C. Lung uptake of lidocaine in healthy volunteers. *Acta Anaesthesiol Scand* 1979;**23**:567–74.

39 Löfström B. Tissue distribution of local anesthetics with special reference to the lung. *Int Anesthesiol Clin* 1978;**16**:53–72.

40 Reynolds F, Laishley R, Morgan B, Lee A. Effect of time and adrenaline on the feto-maternal distribution of bupivacaine. *Br J Anaesth* 1989;**62**:509–14.

41  Kennedy MJ, Heald DL, Bettinger R, David Y. Uptake and distribution of lidocaine in fetal lambs. *Anesthesiology* 1990;**72**:483–9.

42  Abboud TK, Afrasiabi A, Sarkis F *et al.* Continuous infusion epidural analgesia in parturients receiving bupivacaine, chloroprocaine or lidocaine – maternal, fetal and neonatal effects. *Anesth Analg* 1984;**63**:421–8.

43  Denson DD, Coyle DE, Thompson GA, Myers JA. Alpha-1-acid glycoprotein and albumin in human serum bupivacaine binding, *Clin Pharmcol Ther* 1984;**35**:409–15.

44  Pieper JA, Wyman MG, Goldreyer BN, Cannom DS, Slaughter RI, Lalka D. Lidocaine toxicity: effects of total versus free lidocaine concentrations. *Circulation* 1980;**62(III)**:181.

45  Burm AGL, Cohen IMC, van Kleef JW, Vletter AA, Oliemann W, Groen K. Pharmacokinetics of the enantiomers of mepivacaine following intravenous administration of the racemate. *Anesth Analg* 1997;**84**:85–9.

46  Burm AGL, van der Meer AD, van Kleef JW, Zeijlmans PWM, Groen K. Pharmacokinetics of the enantiomers of bupivacaine following intravenous administration of the racemate. *Br J Clin Pharmacol* 1994;**38**:125–9.

47  Seifen AB, Ferrari AA, Seifen EE, Thompson DS, Chapman J. Pharmacokinetics of intravenous procaine infusion in humans. *Anesth Analg* 1979;**58**:382–6.

48  Drayer DE, Lorenzo B, Werns S, Reidenberg MM. Plasma levels, protein binding and elimination data of lidocaine and active metabolites in cardiac patients of various ages. *Clin Pharmacol Ther* 1983;**34**:14–22.

49  Tucker GT, Wiklund L, Berlin-Wahlén A, Mather LE. Hepatic clearance of local anaesthetics in man. *J Pharmacokinet Biopharm* 1977;**5**:111–22.

50  Yoshikawa T. Physiology of aging; impact on pharmacology. *Semin Anesth* 1986;**V**:8–13.

51  Veering BT, Burm AGL, van Kleef JW, Hennis PJ, Spierdijk J. Epidural anesthesia with bupivacaine: effects of age on neural blockade and pharmocokinetics. *Anesth Analg* 1987;**66**:589–94.

52  Bowdle TA, Freund PR, Slattery JT. Age dependent lidocaine pharmacokinetics during lumbar peridural anesthesia with lidocaine hydrocarbonate or lidocaine hydrochloride. *Reg Anesth* 1986;**66**:843–6.

53  Veering BT, Burm AGL, Gladines MPRR, Spierdijk J. Age does not influence the serum protein binding of bupivacaine. *Br J Clin Pharmacol* 1991;**32**:501–3.

54  Bowdle TA, Freund PR, Slattery JT. Propranolol reduces bupivacaine clearance. *Anesthesiology* 1987;**66**:36–8.

55  Noble DW, Smith KJ, Dundas CR. Effects of H$_2$-antagonists on the elimination of bupivacaine. *Br J Anaesth* 1987;**59**:735–7.

56  Palkama VJ, Neuvonen PJ, Olkkola KT. Effect of itraconazole on the pharmacokinetics of bupivacaine enantiomers in healthy volunteers. *Br J Anaesth* 1999;**83**:659–61.

# 2: Toxicity of local anaesthetics associated with regional anaesthesia

PER H ROSENBERG, JEAN-JACQUES ELEDJAM

## Systemic toxicity from unintentional intravascular injection

Unintentional intravascular injection may be the most common cause of systemic local anaesthetic toxicity. All local anaesthetics at high plasma concentrations are toxic to the central nervous system (CNS) and the heart. Therefore, knowledge of recommended maximum doses (Table 2.1) is a primary requisite of the physician who performs the block. In addition, constant alertness for immediate detection of any protoxic symptoms and signs is vital.

If there is a rapid absorption of local anaesthetic into the circulation, toxic CNS symptoms may occur in a relatively standardised order (Fig. 2.1) which, at least in the case of lignocaine (lidocaine), can be related to simultaneously occurring plasma concentrations.[1] On the other hand, if there is direct injection into a blood vessel, the milder CNS symptoms may be bypassed and convulsions and coma may be the symptoms initially observed. In the head and neck region even a small dose (3-4 ml of 0.5% bupivacaine) injected directly into the vertebral or carotid artery may result in convulsions and loss of consciousness. Furthermore, injection into a large vein in the head and neck region, and even into an epidural vein in the thoracic region, may cause direct backflow of a high bolus dose of local anaesthetic into the brain, with immediate toxic consequences.

It is obvious that an acute bolus-type action of a relatively small total dose of a local anaesthetic can produce more severe CNS symptoms than a high peak plasma concentration which has risen slowly. The lungs can take up a considerable amount of local anaesthetic and therefore offer some protection against severe CNS and cardiac toxicity. Postseizure plasma concentrations of local anaesthetics, measured in samples taken from peripheral arteries or veins, usually do not correlate with the toxic symptoms.

Table 2.1 *The clinical use of common local anaesthetics and their recommended maximum doses in adults*

| Local anaesthetic | Concentration (mg/ml) | Clinical use | Onset | Duration | Maximum dose* (mg) |
|---|---|---|---|---|---|
| Lignocaine (lidocaine) | 2.5–10 | Infiltration | Rapid | 1–2 h | 200<br>500 (with adrenaline) |
| | 2.5–5 | Intravenous regional (IVRA) | Rapid | | |
| | 10–15 | Peripheral nerve blocks, e.g. brachial plexus block | Rapid | 1–3 h | |
| | 10–20 | Epidural block | Rapid | 1.5–4 h | |
| | 10–40 | Topical anaesthesia of mucous membranes | Rapid | 0.5–1 h | |
| | 20–50 | Spinal anaesthesia | Rapid | 1–2 h | 60 (higher doses may result in neurotoxicity) |
| Prilocaine | 5–10 | Infiltration | Rapid | 1–2 h | 400<br>600 (with adrenaline) |
| | 2.5–5 | IVRA | Rapid | | |
| | 10–15 | Peripheral nerve blocks | Rapid | 1–3 h | |
| | 10–20 | Epidural block | Rapid | 1–4 h | |
| Mepivacaine | 5–10 | Infiltration | Rapid | 1–2 h | 350<br>500 (with adrenaline) |
| | 10–15 | Peripheral nerve blocks | Rapid | 1–3 h | |
| | 10–20 | Epidural block | Rapid | 1–4 h | |
| | 20–40 | Spinal block | Rapid | 1–2 h | 80 (author's recommendation because of the risk of neurotoxicity) |
| Bupivacaine | 2.5–5 | Infiltration | Rapid | 2–4h | 200<br>200 (with adrenaline) |
| | 2.5–5 | Peripheral nerve blocks | Slow | 4–12 h | |
| | 0.625–2.5 | Obstetric epidural analgesia | Slow-intermediate | 2–4 h | |
| | 2.5–7.5 | Surgical epidural anaesthesia | Intermediate-rapid | 2–5 h | |
| | 1–2.5 | Postoperative epidural analgesia | Intermediate | 2–4 h | |
| | 5–7.5 | Spinal anaesthesia | Rapid | 2–5 h | 22.5 |

| Local anaesthetic | Concentration (mg/ml) | Clinical use | Onset | Duration | Maximum dose* (mg) |
|---|---|---|---|---|---|
| Ropivacaine | 5–10 | Infiltration | Intermediate | 2–8 h | 250 |
|  | 2.5–10 | Peripheral nerve blocks | Slow | 2–8 h | 250 (with adrenaline) |
|  | 1–2 | Obstetric epidural analgesia | Intermediate | 2–4 h |  |
|  | 5–10 | Surgical epidural anaesthesia | Intermediate | 2–5 h |  |
|  | 1–3.75 | Postoperative epidural analgesia | Intermediate | 2–4 h |  |
| Eutectic mixture of lignocaine and prilocaine (EMLA) | 25+25 (mg/g) | Topical anaesthesia, skin | Slow | 1–5 h | 60 g (on intact skin, adult) 2 g (on intact skin, child<1 yr) |
|  |  | Topical, genital mucous membranes | Rapid | 0.25–0.75 h | Recommended doses not available (suggest 50% of skin doses) |
| Procaine | 10 | Topical anaesthesia | Slow | 0.5–1 h | 50 (for mucous membranes, not cornea**) |
|  | 10–20 | Infiltration | Rapid | 1–2 h | 1000 (note allergic potential) |
|  | 10–20 | Peripheral nerve blocks | Slow | 0.5–2 h |  |
|  | 20 | Surgical epidural anaesthesia | Slow | 0.5–2 h |  |
| Chloroprocaine | 10 | Infiltration | Rapid | 0.5–1 h | 800 |
|  | 10–20 | Peripheral nerve blocks | Rapid | 0.5–1 h | 1000 (with adrenaline) |
|  | 10–30 | Surgical epidural anaesthesia | Rapid | 1–2 h |  |
| Amethocaine (tetracaine) | 40 (ointment) (mg/g) | Topical anaesthesia, skin | Slow | 2–4 h | 60 (for skin, not for mucous membranes or cornea) |
|  | 5 | Spinal | Rapid | 2–5 h | 20 |
| Cocaine | 10–40 | Topical | Rapid | 0.5–1 h | Only for ear, nose, throat |

* In adult the recommended dose is for a healthy person (70 kg, 170 cm) and a time period of 4 h.
** In ophthalmology various ester-type local anaesthetics (mainly amethocaine or procaine derivatives) are used for topical corneal and conjunctival anaesthesia.

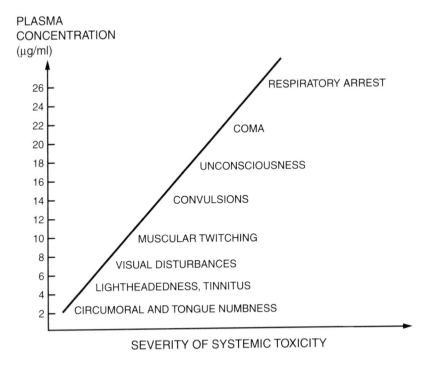

PLASMA
CONCENTRATION
(µg/ml)

Fig 2.1 The relationship between the severity of the CNS toxicity symptoms (x-axis) and plasma concentrations of local anaesthetic (lignocaine) (y-axis)

In order to avoid intravascular injections, injection in small increments (3–5 ml), repeated aspiration attempts, and verbal contact with the patient during local anaesthetic administration should always be routine practice in any local anaesthetic block procedure.

### Rapid absorption and toxicity

The rate of absorption of local anaesthetic into the circulation is determined by tissue vascularity, ambient pH, tissue/plasma drug partition coefficient, and diffusion characteristics. In principle, the absorption is a fixed constant independent of the concentration. At least in man, the concept of constant absorption holds up since it is well established that the local anaesthetic blood (plasma) concentration is proportional to the mass of drug injected.[2]

Capillary wall permeability does not seem to be a limiting factor, as a large drug load is absorbed at the same rate as a small load. Rather, the blood flow through the region is a major determinant and rate-limiting factor in absorption (see Chapter 1). Amide-type local anaesthetics like bupivacaine and lignocaine are absorbed much faster into the circulation from the well-perfused intercostal and epidural spaces than from the poorly perfused subcutaneous fat.

The local perfusion at the injection site can be reduced by adding a vaso-constrictor (usually adrenaline) to the local anaesthetic solution and thus the absorbed local anaesthetic concentration in the bloodstream will be lower (see below). For most local anaesthetics, the recommended maximum dose will be somewhat larger when the solution contains adren-aline (Table 2.1). This is by no means a protection against toxicity from unintentional direct intravascular injection and, in fact, the acute increase of adrenaline concentration in the blood may predispose to cardiac ventric-ular arrhythmias.

In comparison with a direct intravascular injection of local anaesthetics, when even a small dose can cause immediate severe toxicity, systemic toxi-city due to absorption is usually caused by an overdose of local anaesthetic and the symptoms appear after a delay of several minutes (3–15 min).

A continuous infusion of analgesic doses (e.g. 0.125–0.25% bupivacaine, 5–10 ml/h) of local anaesthetic into the epidural or brachial plexus space for the control of postoperative pain, even for two days, does not usually result in systemic toxicity despite the fact that the cumulative dose of bupivacaine may be quite high.[3,4] An increased plasma protein binding of local anaes-thetic, made possible by an increased acute-phase protein synthesis after surgery, will protect the patient from toxicity to a considerable degree.

## Central nervous system toxicity

Central neurotoxicity results from a rapid neuronal desynchronisation at cortical and subcortical brain levels. This is probably associated with a disturbance in the γ-amino butyric acid (GABA) neurotransmitter system at the cellular level, with an inhibition of the chloride channel conduction.[5] These mechanisms form the pharmacological basis of the successful treat-ment of local anaesthetic-induced convulsions with thiopentone, propofol and even diazepam, which act by enhancing GABA-activated chloride flux at the postsynaptic $GABA_A$ receptor.[6]

It has been reported that the incidence of convulsions (severe CNS toxi-city) has ranged from 0.1/1000 in epidural anaesthesia to 0.75–2/1000 in peripheral nerve blocks.[7–9] Convulsions have been described with all local anaesthetics, including the most recent ones, ropivacaine and levobupiva-caine. If there has been no delay in the treatment and hypoxaemia has been avoided, no harmful sequelae have appeared.

## Cardiotoxicity

There is a direct correlation between local anaesthetic potency and toxi-city, making bupivacaine one of the most toxic local anaesthetics. When an inadvertent intravascular injection of a large dose of bupivacaine occurs, there is a great risk of serious cardiac toxicity, i.e. a potent depression of myocardial contractility and a major electrophysiological disturbance. In contrast to systemic toxicity caused by lignocaine and prilocaine, which is primarily expressed in the CNS and only rarely followed by cardiac toxicity, bupivacaine-induced cardiac toxicity may occur simultaneously with the CNS symptoms.

Bupivacaine-induced arrhythmogenic effects result mainly from inhibition of the fast-inward sodium current, $I_{Na}$, which is responsible for the depolarisation of the atria, His bundles, Purkinje cells, and ventricular cells. Bupivacaine binds to the intracellular side of cell membrane sodium channels in their activated state and induces a use-dependent slowing of ventricular conduction velocities, which will facilitate both ventricular conduction defects and ventricular arrhythmias by so-called reentry mechanisms.[10] Clinically observed events are sinus bradycardia, atrioventricular and ventricular blocks, ventricular tachycardia, and ventricular fibrillation. Bupivacaine also impairs the flow of other membrane ion currents, such as slow-inward calcium current, $I_{Ca}$, and delayed potassium current, $I_K$. In addition, bupivacaine induces haemodynamic alterations resulting from the depression of myocardial contractility, mainly due to inhibition of energy metabolism.[11]

Several factors may worsen the cardiotoxicity of bupivacaine, such as hyperkalaemia, hyponatraemia, mild hypothermia, hypoxia, hypercarbia, acidosis, and many different cardioactive medications (calcium channel blockers, β-blocking agents, cibenzoline, disopyramide, clomipramine). Bupivacaine-induced toxic accidents are difficult to treat as both cardiogenic shock and dysrhythmias occur at the same time.

The recent S(–)-enantiomer of 1-propyl-2′,6′-pipecoloxylidide, i.e. ropivacaine, has been shown to offer a higher margin of safety in terms of systemic toxicity.[12,13] Clinically, this potential benefit is often lost by the common use of approximately 1.5 times larger doses of ropivacaine as compared to bupivacaine. Several cases of CNS toxicity caused by ropivacaine have occurred but there are no published reports of dysrhythmias or other cardiotoxic effects from the clinical use of ropivacaine. The S(–)-enantiomer of bupivacaine, levobupivacaine, has been tested and is now available for clinical use. It seems to have an almost identical nerve-blocking effect to racemic bupivacaine but its toxic effects on the CNS and the heart are lower.[14] It may not offer any significant advantage in clinical practice because of its similarity to racemic bupivacaine and the availability of ropivacaine, which is even less toxic.

## Treatment of toxicity

In *mild toxicity* (numbness of the tongue and lips, tinnitus, lightheadedness), no specific treatment is usually necessary. Bedrest for some

20–30 min and reassurance are usually sufficient. When the toxic symptoms are *moderate* (blurring of vision, mild muscular twitching, disorientation), it is safest to keep the patient horizontal, cannulate a peripheral vein for IV fluid (Ringer's solution) administration, give oxygen by mask, and observe the patient for several hours. Usually the symptoms will disapperar within 20-30 min. The patient may become anxious and anxiolytic medication (midazolam 1–2 mg or diazepam 2.5–5 mg IV for adults) may be required. These drugs will also attenuate the muscular overactivity.

If strong *convulsions* (grand mal seizures) develop (the patient usually becomes unconscious), very rapid intervention is necessary. The airways have to be secured and the convulsions stopped and therefore a benzodiazepine is given intravenously (midazolam 2–15 mg or diazepam 5–30 mg for adults, followed by incremental doses as necessary). Alternatively, particularly in the operating room, thiopental 1–3 mg/kg IV or propofol 0.5–2 mg/kg IV is administered. Sometimes endotracheal intubation has to be facilitated by administering suxamethonium 0.25–0.5 mg/kg IV.

Convulsions create hypoxaemia and acidosis and therefore the patient has to be ventilated with 100% oxygen. The magnitude of the metabolic part of the acidosis may be so great that IV sodium bicarbonate may be required (based on arterial blood gas analyses).

The unconsciousness (coma), accentuated by the administered hypnotic drugs, may last for several hours and mechanical ventilation with end-tidal $CO_2$ monitoring will therefore be necessary.

*Cardiotoxicity* of local anaesthetics may occur either by a direct effect on the myocardium[5] and ion channels of the cardiac conduction pathways[15] or by a neurogenic effect mediated by the stimulation of the paraventricular[16] or medullary[17] regions of the brain.

The presence of adrenaline (e.g. adrenaline-containing local anaesthetic solutions), hypoxaemia (unconsciousness, respiratory arrest, convulsions) and acidosis (respiratory arrest, convulsions) will worsen the situation and markedly enhance the risk of mortality, at least when local anaesthetics with high fat solubility and strong protein affinity (such as bupivacaine) are used. Ventricular arrhythmias associated with local anaesthetic cardiotoxicity should not be treated with lignocaine since local anaesthetics potentiate each other's toxicity in an additive manner.[18] Cardiotoxicity without preceding or concomitant CNS toxicity is unlikely. Therefore, the therapy mentioned above, i.e. controlling airways, ventilation with 100% oxygen and IV infusion of Ringer's solution, is the life-saving treatment. In addition, cardiac resuscitation (including manual compression and adrenaline) as well as pharmacological treatment of arrhythmias may be necessary. While the patient convulses it is almost impossible to monitor the ECG and identify the cardiac rhythm so a rapid termination of the convulsions is mandatory.

The best inotropic drug to use in the treatment of cardiogenic shock induced by a potent local anaesthetic is still under debate. Noradrenaline has been found effective in studies in which animals have been resuscitated from asystole,[19] while isoprenaline has been superior to adrenaline[20] and amrinone to placebo[21] in animals resuscitated from non-asystolic local anaesthetic-induced cardiogenic shock. In the case of simultaneous cardiac conduction block, the use of adrenaline should be avoided as it may induce tachycardia, which in turn potentiates the conduction block via the use-dependent effect of the local anaesthetic.

Ventricular fibrillation is treated with a DC shock as usual, but the treatment of other types of arrhythmias must be considered individually. In most cases adequate ventilation and maintenance of good organ perfusion (using cardiac compression as needed, combined with mild inotropic support and adequate fluid loading) for a certain time period (10–30 min) would suffice for cardiac recovery. As mentioned above, the recovery of consciousness may take longer, partly due to the action of the anticonvulsants (sedatives or hypnotics) administered to interrupt the convulsion.

## Other reactions associated with a local anaesthetic block

It is important to realise that not all patient reactions to local anaesthetics or reactions appearing during a block are due to systemic toxicity (Table 2.2). Allergy (anaphylactic reactions) to amide-type local anaesthetics (e.g. lignocaine, mepivacaine, bupivacaine and similar compounds) is extremely rare[22,23] and more often anaphylactic or anaphylactoid skin and airway symptoms are due to additives in the local anaesthetic solution. An extreme skin reaction to the needle stick or some other unpleasant procedure during the performance of the block or soon thereafter may sometimes be difficult to distinguish from an acute allergic reaction, too. Allergy to ester-type local anaesthetics (procaine, amethocaine, and similar compounds) is more common and is often associated with known allergy to agents with a molecular structure related to that of paraaminobenzoic acid.[24] Typically, preservative molecules, for example methylparaben, have this type of basic structure. Delayed-type allergy, appearing after 4–8 hours as urticaria and itching, may be due to the preservative, but other concomitantly administered medication and chemical contacts should also be taken into account.

If allergy is strongly suspected based on earlier reported symptoms, surgery should be postponed and the patient referred for allergy testing.[25] It is advisable to mention in the referral which local anaesthetic was used when the symptoms developed and whether the solution contained any additive (preservative, antioxidant, adrenaline). Also, it is of interest to mention which amide-type local anaesthetic one is planning to use for the intended surgical block.

Readiness to treat an immediate anaphylactic reaction with IV adrenaline

*Table 2.2* Differential diagnosis of reactions which may occur during a local anaesthetic block

| Aetiology | Clinical features | Considerations |
|---|---|---|
| Toxic reaction:<br>– intravascular injection | Immediate convulsions, coma and cardiac toxicity | Coma may develop as initial symptom if a "bolus of blood with high local anaesthetic concentration" reaches the brain |
| – overdosing | Starts after a short delay (2–10 min); gradually appearing toxic symptoms (see Table 2.1) may progress to convulsions | |
| Reactions to adrenaline | Tachycardia, hypertension, headache, anxiety | Varies with dose absorbed and with the type of vasoconstrictor |
| Vasovagal reaction | Rapid onset, bradycardia, hypotension, paleness, fainting | Often already appearing during preparation or at the first needle stick |
| Allergy:<br>– immediate | Anaphylactic reaction, hypotension, bronchospasm, facial and airway swelling | Allergy to amide-type local anaesthetics is rare (other concomitant drugs may be the reason) |
| – delayed | Urticaria | Skin reactions to additives in the local anaesthetic solutions are possible<br>An anaphylactoid skin reaction may cause urticaria |
| High cephalad spread of spinal or epidural anaesthesia | Bradycardia, hypotension, respiratory arrest | Total spinal block may result in coma |
| Shivering | Differential block (thermal sensation nerve fibres are partly blocked), often seen during the recovery phase of epidural or spinal anaesthesia | |
| Acute exacerbation of some disease (e.g. asthma, cardiac insufficency) | Symptoms may resemble those of severe local anaesthetic toxicity | Medical history of the patient is important |

and hydrocortisone, as needed, is a mandatory requisite in any office or hospital unit where local anaesthetic blocks are performed. Milder anaphylactoid symptoms, like itching, may need therapy with an $H_1$-histamine blocker.

Methaemoglobinaemia is a rare complication of local or regional anaesthesia with prilocaine.[26] Ortho-toluidine, an intermediate metabolite of prilocaine, oxidises haemoglobin to methaemoglobin and it has been recommended therefore that the prilocaine dose in adults should not exceed 600 mg. Intravenous methylene blue effectively reduces methaemoglobin back to haemoglobin. Methaemoglobin is also formed from EMLA cream but the risk of hypoxaemia may be real only in infants under 3 months of age.[27]

# Neural damage

Neural damage associated with local anaesthetic blocks may be due to ischaemia (damage to neural blood vessels), trauma (direct destruction by needle) or neurotoxicity (functional disturbance by high concentrations of local anaesthetics). In infiltration and field blocks, trauma to capillaries and small blood vessels cannot be avoided but, fortunately, larger nerve trunks will not usually suffer because they can maintain their blood perfusion and nutrition via an extensive intraneural network of blood vessels. In the case of the spinal neuraxial blocks (spinal or epidural), it is possible to cause ischaemia by injuring an artery feeding the spinal cord or a larger vein which may produce haematoma, pressure, and obstruction of the circulation. Therefore, a meticulous puncturing technique should always be practised and if significant bleeding through the needle occurs during a block procedure, the patient should be observed for symptoms of spinal cord compression. Confirmation of the haematoma by MRI and surgical evacuation of the spinal haematoma within eight hours may prevent irreversible neural damage.[28]

Direct trauma to a nerve may occur by the needle stick, in particular if an injection into a nerve is performed. The chance of permanent damage will increase if the local anaesthetic solution contains adrenaline, which causes sustained intraneural vasoconstriction,[29,30] in addition to an increased intraneural pressure induced by the injectate. Therefore, major nerve blocks should not be performed on patients who are under general anaesthesia and cannot report a paraesthesia from the penetration of the sharp needle tip into a nerve.

In awake patients who report even a weak radiating sensation (paraesthesia) during the performance of a local anaesthetic block, the needle should immediately be withdrawn a few millimetres. Thereafter, a small test dose of the local anaesthetic may be injected in order to confirm the safety of the procedure. One should avoid repeating a peripheral nerve block (needle directed towards a large nerve) at the same site because of the risk of damaging an already anaesthetised nerve. If the initial local anaesthetic conduction block is insufficient, supplemental blocks can be performed at sites closer to or at the region of the surgery, preferably with the aid of a nerve stimulator. Needless to say, knowledge of the anatomy of major nerves is a mandatory requisite of this field of clinical medicine. If bone has been encountered with a sharp bevelled needle, the tip may become barbed[31,32] and the risk of mechanical nerve damage will increase. It is therefore advisable to replace the needle before continuing the blocking procedure.

The currently available commercial local anaesthetic solutions are documented as safe for the neural tissue of the nerve blocks for which they are officially registered (Table 2.1). Therefore, for example, solutions registered for infiltration anaesthesia should not be used for spinal anaesthesia. Most local anaesthetic solutions indicated for infiltration or field blocks contain a preservative (methylparaben) which may be neurotoxic when applied directly to the spinal cord.

Even relatively high concentrations of local anaesthetics (e.g. 4–5% lignocaine) are not directly toxic to peripheral nerves when injected into their close vicinity. The protecting mechanisms include random scattering of the molecules after injection, uptake in surrounding tissues, and absorption into the blood and therefore the majority of the local anaesthetic dose will not reach the nerve axons. On the other hand, when such concentrations are administered into the subarachnoid space, where the protecting mechanisms work more slowly, the risk of neural tissue damage is increased. The spinal anaesthesia-related syndrome called "transient neurological symptoms" (TNSs)[33-35] (see Chapter 8) appears to be associated with the use of hyperbaric concentrated local anaesthetic solutions for the block and, interestingly, with the use of lignocaine in particular, for which there is currently no explanation. The mechanism(s) of TNSs has not yet been completely elucidated and it is possible that technical and mechanical factors (vascular damage, restricted initial spread of the injectate, several puncture attempts) related to the present practice of using very fine needles may also play some role.

## Skeletal muscle toxicity

All local anaesthetics at clinical concentrations are toxic to skeletal muscle tissue.[36] There does not seem to be a clearcut relationship between muscle toxicity and potency of the local anaesthetics but long-acting and strongly protein-bound agents, such as bupivacaine, are suspected to be more damaging than the shorter acting agents. Histological damage in underlying skeletal muscle can be produced experimentally, even after a single subcutaneous injection of bupivacaine. The effect is reversible[36] and even after a week of repeated injections, the muscle tissue regenerates.[37]

Clinically, there are some case reports on permanent muscle damage after local anaesthetic injection directly into muscle tissue.[38,39]

The clinical impact of the skeletal muscle tissue toxicity is generally quite small as long as the potentially damaging agents are not accumulating within or in the vicinity of functionally important groups of muscles. Thus, for example, the delicate eye muscles may be damaged by local anaesthetics injected for para- and retrobulbar eye blocks.[40,41]

1  Scott DB. Evaluation of the toxicity of local anaesthetic agents in man. *Br J Anaesth* 1975;**47**:56–61.

2  Tucker GT, Mather LE. Pharmacokinetics of local anaesthetic agents. *Br J Anaesth* 1975;**47**:213–24.

3  Tuominen M, Haasio J, Hekali R, Rosenberg PH. Continuous interscalene brachial plexus block: clinical efficacy, technical problems and bupivacaine plasma concentrations. *Acta Anaesthesiol Scand* 1989;**33**:84-8.

4  Pere P. The effect of continuous interscalene brachial plexus block with 0.125% bupivacaine plus fentanyl on diaphragmatic motility and ventilatory function. *Reg Anesth* 1993;**18**:93-7.

5  Sawaki K, Ouchi K, Sato T, Kawaguchi M. Some correlations between local anesthetic-induced convulsions and γ-aminobutyric acid in rat spinal cord. *Jpn J Pharmacol* 1991;**56**:327–35.

6  Hales TG, Olsen RW. Basic pharmacology of intravenous induction agents. In: Bowdle TA, Horita A, Kharasch ED, eds. *The pharmacologic basis of anesthesiology*. New York: Churchill Livingstone, 1994:295–306.

7  Brown DL, Ransom DM, Hall JA, Leicht CH. Regional anesthesia and local anesthetic-induced systemic toxicity: seizure frequency and accompanying cardiovascular changes. *Anesth Analg* 1995;**81**:321–8.

8  Auroy Y, Narchi P, Messiah A, Litt L, Rouvier B, Samii K. Serious complications related to regional anesthesia: results of a prospective survey in France. *Anesthesiology* 1997;**87**:479–86.

9  Aromaa U, Lahdensuu M, Cozanitis DA. Severe complications associated with epidural and spinal anaesthesia in Finland 1987–1993. A study based on patient insurance claims. *Acta Anaesthesiol Scand* 1997;**41**:445–52.

10  De la Coussaye J-E, Brugada J, Allessie J. Electrophysiologic and arrhythmogenic effects of bupivacaine. A study with high resolution epicardial mapping in rabbit heart. *Anesthesiology* 1992;**77**:132–41.

11  Eledjam J-J, de la Coussaye J-E *et al.* In vitro study on mechanisms of bupivacaine-induced depression of myocardial contractility. *Anesth Analg* 1989;**69**:732–5.

12  Feldman HS, Arthur GR, Covino BG. Comparative systemic toxicity of convulsant and supraconvulsant doses of intravenous ropivacaine, bupivacaine and lidocaine in the conscious dog. *Anesth Analg* 1989;**69**:794-801.

13  Knudsen K, Beckman Suurküla M, Blomberg S, Sjövall J, Edvardsson N. Central nervous and cardiovascular effects of i.v. infusions of ropivacaine, bupivacaine and placebo in volunteers. *Br J Anaesth* 1997;**78**:507–14.

14  Huang YF, Pryor ME, Mather LE, Veering BT. Cardiovascular and central nervous system effects of intravenous levobupivacaine and bupivacaine in sheep. *Anesth Analg* 1998;**86**:797–804.

15  Reiz S, Nath S. Cardiotoxicity of local anaesthetic agents. Br J Anaesth 1986;**58**:736-46.

16  Covino BG, Wildsmith JAW. Clinical pharmacology of local anesthetic agents. In: Cousins MJ, Bridenbaugh PO, eds. *Neural blockade in clinical anesthesia and management of pain*, 3rd edn. Philadelphia: Lippincott-Raven, 1998:108.

17  Heavner JE. Cardiac dysrhythmias induced by infusion of local anesthetics into the lateral cerebral ventricle of cats. *Anesth Analg* 1986;**65**:133-8.

18  Thomas RD, Behbehani MM, Coyles DE, Denson DD. Cardiovascular toxicity of local anesthetics: an alternative hypothesis. *Anesth Analg* 1986;**65**:444-50.

19  Kyttä J, Heavner JE, Badgewell JM, Rosenberg PH. Cardiovascular and central nervous system effects of co-administered lidocaine and bupivacaine in piglets. *Reg Anesth* 1991;**16**:89-94.

20  Heavner JE, Pitkänen MT, Shi B, Rosenberg PH. Resuscitation from bupivacaine- induced asystole in rats: comparison of different cardioactive drugs. *Anesth Analg* 1995;**80**:1134-9.

21  Buffington CW, Nyström EUM. Treatment of bupivacaine-induced cardiovascular depression in pigs: a comparison of epinephrine and isoproterenol. *Acta Anaesthesiol Scand* 2000;**44**: in press.

22  Lindgren T, Randell T, Suzuki N, Kyttä J, Yli-Hankala A, Rosenberg PH. The effect of amrinone on recovery from severe bupivacaine intoxication in pigs. *Anesthesiology* 1992;**77**:309-15.

23  Adriani J. Drug allergy: local anesthetics. *Anesth Rev* 1984;**11**:14-21.

24  Bridenbaugh PO, Wedel DJ. Complications of local anesthetic neural blockade. In: Cousins MJ, Bridenbaugh PO, eds. *Neural blockade in clinical anesthesia and management of pain*, 3rd edn. Philadelphia: Lippincott-Raven 1998:656.

25  Sindel LJ, de Schazo RD. Accidents resulting from local anesthetics. True or false allergy? *Clin Rev Allergy* 1991;**9**:379-95.

26  Hjelm M, Holmdahl MH. Clinical chemistry of prilocaine and clinical evaluation of methaemoglobin induced by this agent. *Acta Anaesthesiol Scand* 1965;**16(Suppl)**:161-70.

27  Jakobsson B, Nilsson A. Methemoglobinemia associated with prilocaine-lidocaine cream and trimethoprim-sulfamethoxazole. A case report. *Acta Anaesthesiol Scand* 1985;**29**:453-5.

28  Horlocker TT, Heit JA. Low molecular weight heparin: biochemistry, pharmacology, perioperative prophylaxis regimens, and guidelines for regional anesthetic management. *Anesth Analg* 1997;**85**:874-85.

29  Selander D, Månsson LG, Karlsson L, Svanvik J. Adrenergic vasoconstriction in peripheral nerves of the rabbit. *Anesthesiology* 1985;**62**:6-10.

30  Selander D. Peripheral nerve injury after regional anesthesia. In: Finucane BT, ed. *Complications of regional anesthesia*. New York: Churchill Livingstone, 1999:105-15.

31  Stacy GC, Orth D, Hajjar G. Barbed needle and inexplicable paresthesias and trismus after dental regional anesthesia. *Oral Surg* 1994;**77**:585-9.

32  Puolakka R, Jokinen M, Pitkänen M, Rosenberg PH. Comparison of postanesthetic sequelae after clinical use of 27-gauge cutting and noncutting spinal needles. *Reg Anesth* 1997;**22**:521-6.

33  Schneider M, Ettlin T, Kaufmann M, Schumacher P, Urwyler A, Hampl K. Transient neurologic toxicity after hyperbaric subarachnoid anesthesia with 5% lidocaine. *Anesth Analg* 1993;**76**:1154-7.

34 Hiller A, Rosenberg PH. Transient neurological symptoms after spinal anaesthesia with 4% mepivacaine and 0.5% bupivacaine. *Br J Anaesth* 1997;**79**:301–5.

35 Freedman JM, Li D-K, Drasner K, Jaskela MC, Larsen B, Wi S. Transient neurologic symptoms after spinal anesthesia – an epidemiologic study in 1863 patients. *Anesthesiology* 1998;**89**:633–41.

36 Foster AH, Carlson BM. Myotoxicity of local anesthetics and regeneration of the damaged muscle fibers. *Anesth Analg* 1980;**58**:727–36.

37 Kyttä J, Heinonen E, Rosenberg PH, Wahlström T, Gripenberg J, Huopaniemi T. Effects of repeated bupivacaine administration on sciatic nerve and surrounding muscle tissue in rats. *Acta Anaesthesiol Scand* 1986;**30**:625–9.

38 Parris WCV, Dettbarn WD. Muscle atrophy following bupivacaine trigger point injection. *Anesth Rev* 1989;**16**:50–3.

39 Hogan Q, Dotson R, Erickson S, Kettler R, Hogan K. Local anesthetic myotoxicity: a case and a review. *Anesthesiology* 1994;**80**:942–7.

40 Porter JD, Edney DP, McMahon EJ, Burns LA. Extraocular myotoxicity of the retrobulbar anesthetic bupivacaine hydrochloride. *Invest Ophthalm Visual Sci* 1988;**29**:163–74.

41 Hunter DG, Lam GC, Guyton DL. Inferior oblique muscle injury from local anesthesia for cataract surgery. *Ophthalmology* 1995;**102**:501–9.

# 3: Common local anaesthetic blocks

PER H ROSENBERG

## Introduction

In this chapter some of the common local and regional blocks are briefly described. Detailed descriptions of all these blocks can be found in several excellent illustrated textbooks of regional anaesthesia.

Infiltration and most of the peripheral nerve blocks can be performed by all physicians who know the anatomy, equipment, and characteristics of the local anaesthetics. However, certain blocks, for example the brachial plexus block, epidural block, spinal block, and some invasive nerve blocks used in chronic pain therapy, are performed primarily by anaesthesiologists. Special training, manual dexterity, and experience, as well as special knowledge of the therapeutic medications, risks, and complications of such blocks, are required.

In many blocks, large amounts of local anaesthetics are injected and therefore knowledge of the pharmacokinetics and toxicity of these drugs is important (see Chapter 2). Under all circumstances, great attention must be paid to preventing and detecting accidental intravascular injection of a local anaesthetic.

## Infiltration block, field block, and peripheral nerve blocks

### Infiltration block

Infiltration of local anaesthetic into the skin (Fig. 3.1) and underlying structures for various painful procedures, such as suturing of a wound or performing a transcutaneous puncture, is a common procedure which should be mastered by all physicians. For the infiltration of large areas it is preferable to use long needles so that the number of punctures can be kept to a minimum; for instance, the 22 G spinal needle is well suited for such a

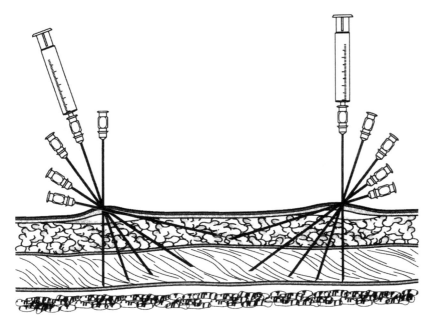

Fig. 3.1    Fan-like infiltration of the various layers of the skin with local anaesthetic for surgical incision. In order to shorten the delay of complete sensory block of the skin, i.e. time to incision, it is important also to infiltrate the most superficial layer. If large amounts (volumes) are needed, adrenaline (5 µg/ml) should be added to the solution

purpose. On the other hand, if only a small area needs to be infiltrated, the smallest possible needle, of sufficient length, is chosen.

In order to block relevant terminal nerves and nerve endings it is usually necessary to inject relatively large volumes of the local anaesthetic solution. Since systemic toxicity is directly related to the total dose injected, it is necessary to use as dilute solutions of the local anaesthetic as possible when large areas have to be anaesthetised. Thus, instead of using a 1% lignocaine solution, a 0.5% solution will normally provide adequate anaesthesia (the onset may take a few minutes longer). The recommended maximum dose of the local anaesthetic (see Table 2.1, pp. 23–24) should not be exceeded.

If possible, adrenaline (5 µg/ml) is added to prolong the action of the block, as well as to achieve vasoconstriction and a bloodless surgical field, when necessary. When large volumes of adrenaline-containing local anaesthetic solution are used, the administered adrenaline dose must also be considered. It has been suggested that the amount of adrenaline should not exceed 1.5 µg/kg in a period of 10 min; for example, when a solution containing 5 µg/ml (1:200 000) adrenaline is infiltrated in a 70 kg patient, no more than 21 ml should be administered.[1] Over a period of one hour, no more than 8 µg/kg of adrenaline should be given. Some commercial local anaesthetic solutions contain 10 µg/ml of adrenaline and may be used in blocks of the mucosa of the mouth region. Due to the risk of ischaemic tissue damage, it is not advisable to use adrenaline-containing solutions in blocks of the most peripheral parts of the body, such as the nose, ear lobes, fingers, toes, and penis.

Despite some confusion regarding the reported variability of the vasoactivity of local anaesthetics between animals and man, as well as between different vessel groups, a simplified clinical extrapolation can be recommended. In cases where the use of adrenaline would be contraindicated (e.g. increased risk of cardiac arrhythmias) but some vasoconstriction is desired, mepivacaine would be a good choice for infiltration or field blocks of short or intermediate duration.[2] Ropivacaine, which has consistently produced some degree of vasoconstriction or does not produce vasodilatation in experimental studies,[3,4] would be a good choice for blocks of long duration.

An infiltration block commonly performed by non-anaesthesiologists is the *haematoma block* for the manipulation of a Colles' fracture. In this block 10–15 ml of a 1–2% solution of lignocaine or prilocaine (without adrenaline) is injected directly into the haematoma around the fracture at the distal head of the radius. The injection site is, in fact, identified by aspirating blood into the syringe. This is by no means an ideal regional anaesthetic technique because it often produces inadequate analgesia[5] and there is an increased risk of systemic toxicity due to rapid vascular absorption. Its popularity is based on the fact that it is easy to perform and less time consuming than the more analgesically adequate alternatives, i.e. brachial plexus block or intravenous regional anaesthesia (IVRA), which also would require the presence of an anaesthesiologist.

## Field block

A field block is a special modification of the infiltration block in which the varying subcutaneous course of the cutaneous nerves is taken into account. In particular, when the intended surgery requires good identification of the anatomical structures, it is necessary that the needle puncture and instillation of local anaesthetic are performed outside the surgical site. Because the innervation of the skin overlaps, to a great extent, a rhombus-shaped local anaesthetic barrier will often be injected around the incision site (Fig. 3.2). If the estimated surgery is long (>1 h) adrenaline may be added to the local anaesthetic solution. Supplemental

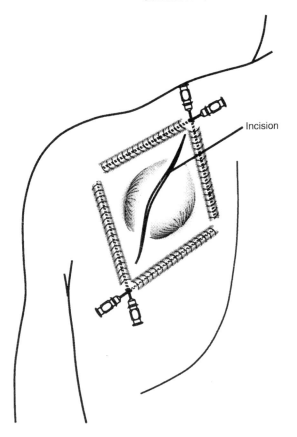

Incision

Fig. 3.2   Local anaesthetic infiltration of the skin from two puncture points to surround the site of skin incision or for the excision of a small superficial tumour

local anaesthetic infiltration during the course of surgery, when required, is not a problem as long as the maximum recommended dose of the local anaesthetic is kept in mind.

## Peripheral nerve block (block of major nerves or nerve trunks)

A peripheral nerve block is placed proximal to the site of the scheduled painful procedure or the site of pain. These blocks can be accomplished either by injecting local anaesthetic according to anatomical landmarks (e.g. intercostal nerve block), searching for paraesthesia with the needle tip (e.g. some techniques of brachial plexus block) or by using a special nerve stimulator connected to the needle (e.g. femoral nerve block, some techniques of brachial plexus block).

### Intercostal nerve block

This is used to treat pain due to fractured ribs and to produce unilateral analgesia of the thorax or abdomen (Fig. 3.3). The transcutaneous puncture is performed as posteriorly as possible, most often in the posterior axillary line, at the relevant intercostal level. At this injection site and at sites still closer to the spine, the injected local anaesthetic solution can spread by flow and diffusion longitudinally beneath the parietal pleura to the adjacent one or two intercostal spaces.[6] In this way the number of needle sticks and the risk of pneumothorax can be reduced.

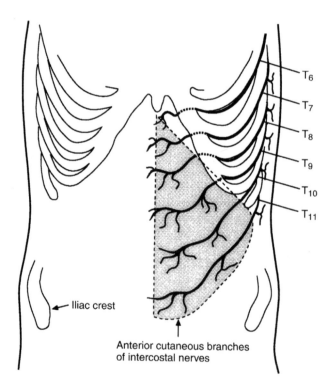

Fig. 3.3    Block of the intercostal nerves is usually quite predictable as the nervous distribution follows the corresponding rib. Note that the outer layers of the abdominal wall from the level of the xiphoid to that of the iliac crests are innervated by the anterior cutaneous branches of the lowest intercostal nerves (the 12th intercostal nerve is not depicted here)

Preferably, a short-bevelled needle is used, first establishing contact with the lower edge of the relevant rib, then "walking" the needle tip below the edge and advancing the needle carefully about 3 mm into the intercostal groove (Fig. 3.4). After careful aspiration to exclude interpleural or intravascular puncture, local anaesthetic is injected in fractions. A long-acting local anaesthetic should always be used, for example 0.5% bupivacaine or 0.75% ropivacaine, 15 ml if there is only one injection site or, alternatively, 5 ml at each level in the case of multiple rib fractures or a large pain area.

Rare complications of intercostal nerve block include pneumothorax, systemic toxicity due to direct intravascular injection or rapid intravascular

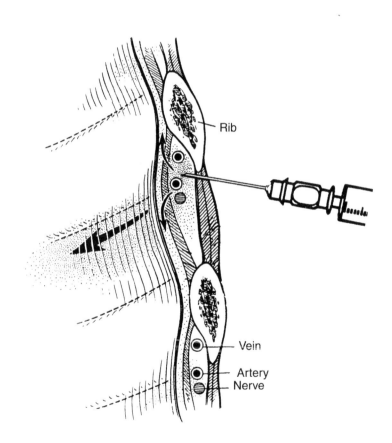

Fig. 3.4   Needle position in a percutaneous intercostal nerve block. The needle is "walked" below the lower edge of the rib and advanced carefully into the intercostal space. In order to avoid perforation of the parietal pleura, a short-bevelled block needle should be used

absorption, and hypotension due to concomitant blockade of the adjacent paravertebral sympathetic trunk.

*Brachial plexus block*

This is used for surgical anaesthesia and for the treatment of various painful conditions of the upper extremity. There are several modifications (approaches) of the brachial plexus block and, in principle, they can be divided into supraclavicular techniques and infraclavicular techniques according to the puncture site (Fig. 3.5). The most common supraclavicular technique is probably the interscalene brachial plexus block, with its modifications,[7] and the most common infraclavicular technique is the axillary brachial plexus block. The interscalene brachial plexus block is used mainly for surgery and the treatment of pain in the shoulder and the brachium (it can also be used for the whole upper extremity),[8] while the

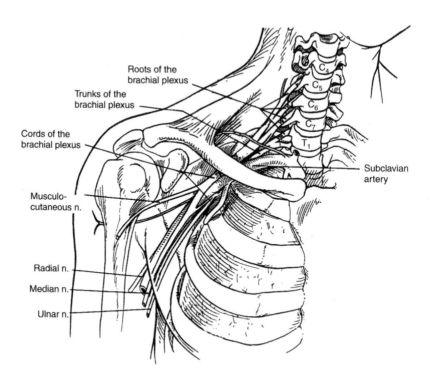

Fig. 3.5  The brachial plexus can be reached by a block needle at different sites above (supraclavicular approaches) or below (infraclavicular approaches) the clavicle. In the supraclavicular brachial plexus block approaches, the phrenic nerve, emanating from C3–5, will always be blocked too

axillary brachial plexus block is used for surgery and the treatment of pain of the hand and the antebrachium.

Some older anaesthesiologists identify the plexus by touching the nerves with the needle tip, i.e. searching for paraesthesia. The modern and more preferable technique utilises nerve stimulation to find the correct injection site. Specially designed plexus-blocking sets include a short-bevelled needle which can be connected to a nerve stimulator and some sets contain a plastic introducer cannula and catheter for continuous blocks. The brachial plexus is identified by the nerve stimulator technique, using as low a current as possible (<0.5 mA at 2 Hz). In adult patients, 40–50 ml of 1% ligno-caine, mepivacaine or prilocaine is injected for short-lasting (<2 h) surgery, while 0.5% bupivacaine or 0.75% ropivacaine can be used for longer lasting (<6 h) surgery. In clinical practice, however, when long surgery is expected, a catheter is inserted into the plexus space to allow for the possibility of continuing the block, when necessary, as well as to provide good postoper-ative analgesia.[9]

The brachial plexus block with the shorter acting local anaesthetics may be intensified and prolonged by adding adrenaline (5 μg/ml) to at least part of the solution (maximum 1.5 μg/kg/10 min). In the case of the long-acting local anaesthetics, adrenaline inclusion is not necessary other than, perhaps, in the first 5–10 ml of the injectate for the immediate detection of a possible intravascular injection.

Complications of brachial plexus blocks are common to all techniques with regard to toxicity (40–50 ml of any 0.5–1% local anaesthetic solution injected into a vein can produce severe systemic toxicity) and needle-induced damage, both of which are rare. These complications can be avoided almost completely by adopting a careful needle-handling technique and injecting the local anaesthetic solution in small, 5 ml fractions. The supraclavicular techniques always cause a block of the ipsilateral phrenic nerve which results in ipsilateral diaphragmatic paralysis for as long as the block is active.[10] In those supraclavicular block techniques (modifications) where the puncture site is close to the clavicle, there is a small risk of pneu-mothorax which may exclude the use of such modified plexus blocks for day surgery patients (see also Chapter 9).

*Femoral and sciatic nerve blocks*

These blocks are used for surgery of the lower extremity in cases where epidural or spinal anaesthesia is not applicable, for example due to an infection of the skin of the lumbar region. They are also utilised for the control of postoperative pain in regions corresponding to their innervations, either as intermittent injections or as continuous catheter techniques.

Both the femoral and sciatic nerves can be identified by the nerve stimulator technique. The needles and sets used for the brachial plexus block can also be utilised for the block of the femoral nerve and for the popliteal approach of the sciatic nerve block. On the other hand, for the sciatic nerve blockade at the hip level, by the anterior or posterior approach, a longer (10–15 cm), short-bevelled nerve stimulator needle has to be used.

For the *femoral block*, the femoral nerve is localised immediately lateral to the femoral artery, just below the inguinal ligament. A nerve stimulator needle is carefully advanced cephalad at an angle of about 30°. With a stimulation current of 0.5 mA or lower, a motor response is elicited in the rectus femoris muscle, including a patellar movement. The femoral nerve is outside the femoral sheath, separated from the femoral artery and femoral vein by the iliopsoas fascia. Therefore, it is important that the motor response is obtained by using a low stimulating current which is an indication of the needle tip being located near or even directly on the nerve. If only a single injection is to be made, such as in the case of short-lasting minor surgery in areas covered by femoral nerve innervation, 15–20 ml of 1% lignocaine, 0.5% bupivacaine or 0.75% ropivacaine is injected. If, on the other hand, the block is used for postoperative pain relief after total knee arthroplasty, initially a catheter set should be used and a cannula or a catheter inserted along the femoral nerve. Continuous analgesia can be provided by a continuous infusion of, for example, 0.25% bupivacaine or 0.375% ropivacaine at a rate of 5–10 ml/h or by intermittent injections of the single-injection dose of bupivacaine or ropivacaine, when required but not more frequently than at about 5–6-hour intervals.

By threading a catheter along the femoral nerve all the way to the level of the lumbar plexus divisions (near the spine), it is possible to produce a so-called "three-in-one block" (femoral nerve, obturator nerve, and lateral femoral cutaneous nerve) by injecting a relatively large volume (15–20 ml) of local anaesthetic.[11] The optimal catheter position cannot usually be guaranteed without the aid of a special guidewire (the Seldinger technique).

The *sciatic nerve block* can be used alone for surgery of the foot and ankle, except in the medial part of the ankle and the foot which is innervated by the saphenous nerve (division of the femoral nerve). It can also be used for the treatment of pain due to broken toes or broken calcaneus. For amputation of the leg below the knee, it is also necessary to block the femoral nerve. Among the various approaches to sciatic nerve block, only the popliteal technique is described here because technically it is relatively easy to perform and clinically it is quite useful.

High up in the popliteal fossa, the sciatic nerve is divided into the tibial nerve and the deep peroneal nerve. A plexus catheter set with nerve stimulator needle is used.[12] With the patient prone, the puncture is performed at a point high up in the popliteal fossa, in normal-sized adults about 10 cm above the popliteal skin crease (Fig. 3.6). The conducting needle is introduced cephalad at an angle of about 45° to the skin. Using a stimulating

Fig. 3.6 The skin puncture site for the popliteal sciatic nerve block, approximately 10 cm from the popliteal skin crease in a normal-sized adult. The nerve stimulator needle is directed cephalad at a 45° angle for the identification of the point of the sciatic nerve where it divides into the tibial nerve and the common peroneal nerve (reproduced with permission from Singelyn FJE. *Tech Reg Anesth Pain Manag* 1998; **2:** 90–5)

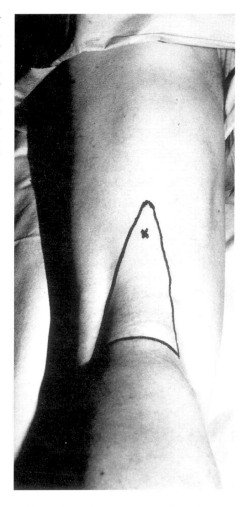

current of 0.5–1 mA, a visible twitch of the foot (plantarflexion) is observed. For a single-injection block, depending on the duration of surgery, either 20–30 ml of 1% mepivacaine or 0.5% bupivacaine is injected. For longer lasting surgery and for the control of postoperative pain, a catheter is introduced with the aid of a guidewire. Either intermittent boluses or a continuous infusion of local anaesthetic are administered, as indicated. Continuous infusion analgesia can be provided by 0.25% bupivacaine or 0.375% ropivacaine at a rate of 5–10 ml/h. In order to reduce the degree of motor block and provide sufficient analgesia, a combination of 0.125% bupivacaine with sufentanil 0.1 µg/ml and clonidine 1 µg/ml has been found efficacious.[12]

Complications of the femoral and sciatic nerve blocks are very rare. Due to the large bolus dose employed in single-injection blocks, systemic toxicity is naturally a risk to be considered.

*Ankle block*

The *ankle block* is an effective peripheral nerve block for surgery of the foot. By blocking all the innervation of the foot provided by the distal divisions of both the sciatic nerve (sural nerve, tibial nerve, deep and superficial peroneal nerves) and the femoral nerve (saphenous nerve) at the level of the ankle (malleoli), complete anaesthesia can be achieved. Therefore, this block is an excellent regional anaesthetic technique for surgery of both the sole and the dorsum of the foot.

A tourniquet around the ankle may be applied but because the site of the tourniquet cuff will not be anaesthetised, the cuff cannot be kept inflated for longer than approximately 30 min. Naturally, this block should not be performed if the skin at the ankle level is infected. However, in the case of an infection or gangrene peripheral to the ankle (e.g. in the toes), the block may be used.

The ankle block can be performed using three separate needle punctures, i.e. the anterior innervation is blocked via one puncture (Fig. 3.7). No nerve stimulator is required. The sural nerve is blocked behind the lateral malleolus (needle stick 1) and the posterior tibial nerve behind the medial malleolus (needle stick 2). By using a long (9–10 cm) needle the rest of the relevant innervation can be blocked via one skin puncture (needle stick 3): the deep peroneal nerve between the extensor hallucis longus muscle and the anterior tibial muscle, and the saphenous nerve (in front of the medial malleolus) as well as the cutaneous branches of the superficial peroneal nerve (in front of the ankle). Alternatively, all five sites can be approached separately using thin short-bevelled needles. For each nerve group, 3–5 ml of 0.5% bupivacaine or 0.75% ropivacaine may be injected. When only three sticks are made, the volume injected through the needle inserted in the front of the ankle should be 6–10 ml, i.e. the total volume should be 15–20 ml.

Rare complications of the ankle block include haematoma and transient neuropathy. Both are avoidable by applying the needles carefully.

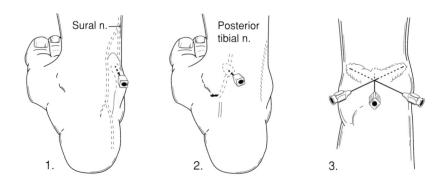

Fig. 3.7 An ankle block, which provides anaesthesia of the whole foot, can be performed via three skin punctures. 1. Block of the sural nerve behind the lateral malleolus. 2. Block of the posterior tibial nerve behind the medial malleolus. 3. Block of the peroneal nerve divisions and the saphenous nerve division

# Central (neuraxial) nerve blocks

## Epidural anaesthesia

The epidural (peridural) space is the region between the dura mater and the ligaments and periosteum that line the vertebral canal. It extends from the foramen magnum to the sacrococcygeal membrane. This is a potential space, normally completely filled with loose adipose tissue, connective tissue strands and bands, blood vessels, and lymphatics. Local anaesthetic and other drugs injected into the epidural space can enter the cerebrospinal fluid (CSF) by penetrating directly through the dura mater and the arachnoid. The main nerve-blocking action results from the spread of the solution laterally to the nerve root sleeve (dural cuff) region where the local anaesthetic is taken up into the CSF and into the spinal cord.[13]

Epidural anaesthesia is usually subdivided into three categories depending on the site of injection: thoracic epidural, lumbar epidural, and caudal block. Cervical epidural analgesia (not anaesthesia) is sometimes applied in the treatment of severe pain in the lower cervical and upper thoracic dermatomal levels. Thoracic epidural anaesthesia is only very rarely indicated as the sole technique for abdominal surgery. Instead, nowadays, combination with general anaesthesia is very common for most types of upper abdominal surgery, allowing postoperative pain to be controlled by this regional anaesthetic technique. Similarly, lumbar epidural anaesthesia is most often used in combination with general anaesthesia, in particular for abdominal surgery. For non-abdominal surgery below the umbilicus (urological, gynaecological, orthopaedic), lumbar epidural anaesthesia alone is often sufficient.

For the epidural puncture, the most common type of needle is the Tuohy needle with a curved Huber point and a bevel facing sideways (Fig. 3.8). By using relatively large needles in adults, 16 G and 18 G, the various tissue layers penetrated by the needle can be easily felt. The curved tip allows smooth insertion of a plastic (usually nylon or polyurethane) catheter into the epidural space. Although the immediate direction taken by the catheter can be guided by the Tuohy needle, the location of the tip after passage of the catheter further than 3–4 cm into the epidural space may be difficult to predict. The catheters have several openings (side holes) near the rounded "atraumatic" tip. In order to minimise the risk of accidental intravascular placement or dural penetration of the catheter, special catheters with flexible plastic tips or spring wires distal to the catheter orifice have been developed (see Chapter 5). Straight-tip short-bevelled needles (e.g. the Crawford-type needle) are rarely used because of the relatively greater risk of a dural tap, at least when the puncture is made in the midline.

47

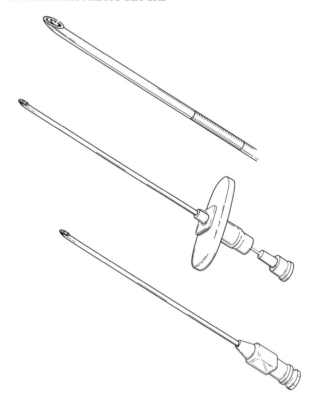

Fig. 3.8   Typical Tuohy needles used for epidural anaesthesia. Note the curved tip, which allows easy introduction of a plastic catheter. The wing on the needle in the middle can be held by both hands when slowly advancing the needle

In principle, any of the currently marketed local anaesthetics could be used for epidural anaesthesia. It is recommended that a test dose of local anaesthetic (to detect an inadvertent subarachnoid injection) mixed with adrenaline (to detect an inadvertent intravascular injection) is first injected. Commonly, the test dose in adults consists of 3 ml of 0.5% bupivacaine mixed with 15 μg of adrenaline. The patient is observed for 3–5 min for a possible developing spinal block (in the event of dural perforation) or a marked increase in heart rate (in the event of intravascular injection) before commencing administration of the main dose of the epidural local anaesthetic.

It is suggested that in short procedures in adults, 15–20 ml of 1.5% lignocaine or mepivacaine may be used, remembering that the maximum recommended dose of lignocaine without adrenaline is only 200 mg

(350 mg for mepivacaine). For longer surgical procedures, catheter tech-niques are preferred, and for the initial block 15–20 ml of 0.5% bupiva-caine or 0.75% ropivacaine is injected. When the extent of the initial block has been established (e.g. testing by needle pinprick or with an ice cube on the skin), usually within 30–45 min, the possible need for sup-plemental doses can be determined. Some anaesthesiologists prefer to mix 2% lignocaine at various proportions with 0.75% bupivacaine or 1% ropivacaine in order to speed up the onset of the block. The fact remains that in controlled studies, the saving in onset time by using mixtures of local anaesthetics (short-acting + long-acting) is clinically insignificant.

Lumbar epidural analgesia is commonly used for the control of obstetric pain. The epidural test dose is adrenaline free and may consist of 7.5–10 mg of bupivacaine or 10–12.5 mg of ropivacaine. The main intermittent doses are selected individually and varying volumes (5–10 ml) of 0.06–0.125% bupivacaine or 0.1–0.2% ropivacaine are employed. In many centres small amounts of fentanyl (1–3 μg/ml) or sufentanil (0.2–0.4 μg/ml) are added to the dilute local anaesthetic solutions. For caesarean section, in a non-emer-gency situation, the preplaced epidural catheter can be utilised and 0.5% bupivacaine or 0.75% ropivacaine, at intermittent boluses of 5 ml, may be administered until the spread of analgesia reaches the fourth thoracic dermatomal level.

Perhaps more commonly today, a combined spinal and epidural (CSE) technique is used. When the epidural catheter is already in place and has been employed for obstetric analgesia, a separate subarachnoid puncture is made via an adjacent lower vertebral interspace. However, when the patient is scheduled directly for a caesarean section, the modern "single-interspace" needle-through-needle CSE technique (Fig. 5.5, p. 74) has become the method of choice.[14] First, an epidural Tuohy needle is placed into the epidural space serving as introducer for the spinal needle. When the spinal anaesthetic dose has been injected and the spinal needle with-drawn, an epidural catheter is inserted via the Tuohy needle. Hyperbaric 0.5% bupivacaine, 1.5–2 ml, will be injected subarachnoidally which produces a surgical block much more rapidly than that achieved by the epidural route. CSE can be performed directly so that in the same punc-ture session a double-interspace techniqe is used. An epidural catheter is placed first and the spinal block is then performed in an adjacent caudad interspace.

Caudal anaesthesia (performed by puncturing the sacrococcygeal liga-ment) in adults is rarely used for surgical anaesthetic purposes. Instead, caudal analgesia is used for diagnostic and therapeutic blocks in chronic pain. In children, the caudal block has attained a routine status in many institutions as a postoperative analgesic method performed at the end of surgery to the lower part of the body.[15]

In the treatment of postoperative pain 0.06–0.25% bupivacaine or 0.1–0.375% ropivacaine may be infused via an epidural catheter, in adults at a rate of 4–10 ml/h. Currently, an opioid (morphine, fentanyl, sufentanil) is added to the epidural solution to diminish the local anaesthetic-induced motor block and maintain an adequate quality of analgesia.[16]

Complications of epidural anaesthesia include puncture-related, toxic, circulatory, and infectious reactions.[17] Fortunately, the incidence of complications is low; for example, that of spinal haematoma is less than 1 in 150 000.[18] Obviously, neuraxial blocks should not be performed in fully anticoagulated patients because severing of small blood vessels by the needle or catheter would easily lead to a spinal haematoma. Low-molecular weight heparin (LMWH) is nowadays used for thromboprophylaxis in patients undergoing major orthopaedic surgery, as well as other major surgery after which the patient may be immobile for some days. As a practical recommendation, the epidural block should not be performed within 10–12 hours after the last LMWH (enoxaparin, dalteparine) dose and the first dose after the epidural puncture (catheterisation) should not be given within two hours. Also, the removal of a catheter should not be performed within 10–12 hours after an LMWH dose and the next dose should not be given within two hours.

Epidural infections and abscesses are also rare and may be due to a systemic infection or to contamination from the skin (Staphylococcus).[17]


## Spinal anaesthesia

A spinal block is performed caudad to the second lumbar vertebral process, usually in the L3–4 interspace. A small dose of local anaesthetic is distributed in the lumbar portion of the CSF and the primary nerve-blocking action occurs at the level of the nerve roots near the site of injection. In principle, therefore, anaesthetising the lower part of the body is most predictable while the cephalad spread of the block (analgesia or anaesthesia) is unpredictable. By using local anaesthetic solutions made hyperbaric ("heavy") relative to the CSF by adding glucose (5–10%), the spread of a spinal block can be adjusted, to some extent, by changing the position of the patient as needed.

A subarachnoid puncture can be performed with the patient in the horizontal side position or in the sitting position, with a flexed back comfortably but firmly supported by an assistant. For the patient it is more comfortable to be lying because this may prevent dizziness and fainting in an anxious patient when the procedure is time consuming due to multiple puncture attempts.

The disinfected puncture site is infiltrated with a small dose of local anaesthetic. Directional stability and reduction of tissue coring by the spinal needle can be provided by first placing a 30 mm 20 G introducer needle to the depth of the interspinous ligaments. The spinal needle is then advanced carefully via the introducer through the ligamentum flavum, the epidural space, dura mater, and pia arachnoid into the CSF. Thin 25–27 G styletted spinal needles, with either a cutting tip or a non-cutting, pencil-point tip, are used (see Fig. 5.1, p. 67 and Fig. 5.3, p. 68). The pencil-point tips are advantageous in the sense that the risk of post-dural puncture headache (PDPH) can be lowered. These needles also cause less damage to the fibres of the dura than the cutting needle tips and less leakage of CSF through the dura.[18] In adults the needle shaft length should be at least 9 cm so that the whole side opening on the pencil-point tips will reach the subarachnoid space in a relatively big patient. For extremely big (obese) patients, it is advisable to utilise the spinal needle (11–13 cm) from a combined spinal epidural (CSE) set with the epidural needle as introducer. On the other hand, for children shorter (2.5–5 cm) 24–27 G spinal needles are available.

When the needle tip orifice is assumed to be in the subarachnoid space, the stylet is withdrawn and usually a free flow of CSF can be seen in a few seconds. With the thinnest needles, for example 29 G, there is often no free CSF flow but a correct needle tip position may be ascertained by easy aspiration and reinjection of CSF with a small syringe. Thereafter, the syringe with the prescheduled anaesthetic dose is attached to the needle, 0.2–0.5 ml of CSF is aspirated into the syringe and this, together with the local anaesthetic, is injected. Again, after injection the aspiration/reinjection of CSF is repeated to verify the success of the technical performance of the spinal block.

The needle is removed and the patient is placed in the desired position on the operating table, depending on the site of surgery and the baricity of the local anaesthetic solution. Although baricity may be considered the most important factor determining the spread of the spinal block, the elimination of the long-acting local anaesthetic bupivacaine from the CSF is relatively slow and a change in patient position even after 45–60 min may cause a secondary spread of the block.

All local anaesthetics have in the past been used for clinical spinal anaesthesia, including cocaine.[19] Nowadays, only local anaesthetics which are officially registered and are free of antioxidants and preservatives can be used for spinal anaesthesia. This may vary from country to country but in recent years those most commonly used have been the amide-type local anaesthetics bupivacaine and lignocaine as well as the ester-type local anaesthetics amethocaine (tetracaine) and procaine. Bupivacaine has been found to be most useful in both long-lasting anaesthesia for hip replacement and short-lasting day surgery anaesthesia for knee arthroscopy. In adults, doses of 15–20 mg of plain (slightly hypobaric) 0.5% bupivacaine will provide anaesthesia of the lower extremities for 2–5 hours, while a dose of 7.5–10 mg of a hyperbaric solution will anaesthetise the hip region for only about 60–90 min.

For many years lignocaine 1.5–5%, isobaric or hyperbaric, was the most popular spinal anaesthetic for surgeries of short duration (<1.5 hours). However, due to the transient neurologic symptoms syndrome (TNSs; see Chapter 8), lignocaine is no longer favoured in spinal anaesthesia. A hyperbaric 4% solution of mepivacaine, which has been registered for spinal anaesthesia in some countries, has also been associated with TNSs as frequently as lignocaine (incidence approximately 30%).

Amethocaine is mixed with distilled water, cerebrospinal fluid or glucose to make a 1% solution, either hypobaric, isobaric or hyperbaric, respectively. A dose of 10–15 mg amethocaine produces surgical anaesthesia of the lower extremities for 1–3 hours and the duration can be prolonged approximately by an hour by adding adrenaline (0.2–0.3 mg) to the solution.

Procaine is used in some centres as a 5% solution mixed with distilled water, cerebrospinal fluid or glucose. Doses of 100–200 mg in adults produce short-lasting anaesthesia (<60 min) of the lower part of the body.

Spinal anaesthesia is commonly used for surgery of the lower part of the body, perhaps most typically for orthopaedic surgery. Operations for reconstruction of arteries of the lower extremities, varicose veins of the lower extremities, inguinal hernia, anal haemorrhoids, prostate hypertrophy, diseases of vagina/uterus, etc. are performed under spinal anaesthesia. Because of a very low risk of PDPH from the use of thin pencil-point spinal needles, spinal anaesthesia has also become more and more popular as a routine technique in day surgery. Caesarean sections can be performed under spinal anaesthesia but nowadays the CSE technique (see Fig. 3.9) has become the standard anaesthetic technique for a non-emergency caesarean section.

Continuous spinal anaesthesia, by introducing a catheter into the subarachnoid space, is a useful technique in long-lasting orthopaedic operations of the lower extremities and the catheter can also be used for continuous postoperative spinal analgesia.[20] In elderly patients, in whom PDPH is less of a risk, epidural catheters (20–24 G) can safely be utilised as spinal catheters.

Complications of spinal anaesthesia are, in part, similar in quality and frequency to those of epidural anaesthesia. Systemic toxicity does not occur because of the small dose injected.

In the case of thromboprophylaxis with LMWH, the same precautions as were mentioned under epidural anaesthesia have to be considered.

Because a needle and drug are introduced directly into the CNS special attention must be paid to factors which guarantee sterility and to the technical performance. Meningitis after spinal anaesthesia has been reported as a rare complication.[17] PDPH cannot be avoided totally and with the use of thin pencil-point spinal needles, the incidence in inpatients is approximately 1% and in outpatients it is a little more frequent. Most of these postural-dependent headaches are self-limiting and will vanish in 4–7 days. If indicated, immediate relief can usually be provided by injecting autologous blood (approximately 10 ml), under sterile conditions, into the patient's epidural space near the previous site of the dural puncture (epidural blood patch).

1  Raj PP, Pai U, Rawal N. Techniques of regional anesthesia in adults. In: Raj PP, ed. *Clinical Practice of regional anesthesia*. New York: Churchill Livingstone, 1991:272.

2  Guinard J-P, Carpenter RL, Morell RC. Effect of local anesthetic concentration on capillary blood flow in human skin. *Reg Anesth* 1992;**17**:317–21.

3  Kopacz DJ, Carpenter RL, Mackey DC. Effect of ropivacaine on cutaneous capillary blood flow in pigs. *Anesthesiology* 1989;**71**:69–74.

4  Dahl JB, Simonsen L, Mogensen T, Henriksen JH, Kehlet H. The effect of 0.5% ropivacaine on epidural blood flow. *Acta Anaesthesiol Scand* 1990;**34**:308–10.

5  Haasio J. Cubital nerve block vs. haematoma block for the manipulation of Colles' fracture. *Ann Chir Gynaec* 1990;**79**:168–71.

6  Nunn JF, Slavin G. Posterior intercostal nerve blockade for pain relief after cholecystectomy. *Br J Anaesth* 1980;**52**:253–9.

7  Haasio J, Rosenberg PH. Continuous supraclavicular brachial plexus anesthesia. *Tech Reg Anesth Pain Manag* 1997;**1**:157–62.

8  Winnie AP. *Plexus anesthesia, vol. I*. Fribourg: Mediglobe SA, 1990.

9  Tuominen M, Haasio J, Hekali R, Rosenberg PH. Continuous interscalene brachial plexus block: clinical efficacy, technical problems, and bupivacaine plasma concentrations. *Acta Anaesthesiol Scand* 1989;**33**:128–31.

10  Pere P, Pitkänen M, Rosenberg PH *et al*. Effect of continuous interscalene brachial plexus block on diaphragm motion and on ventilatory function. *Acta Anaesthesiol Scand* 1992;**36**:138–41.

11  Postel J, März P. Die kontinuerliche Blockade des Plexus lumbalis ("3-in-1 block") in der perioperativen Schmerztherapie. (abstract in English) *Regional-Anaesthesie* 1984;**7**:140–3.

12  Singelyn FJ, Aye F, Gouverneur JM. Continuous popliteal sciatic nerve block: an original technique to provide postoperative analgesia after foot surgery. *Anesth Analg* 1998;**84**:383–6.

13  Cousins MJ, Veering BT. Epidural neural blockade. In: Cousins MJ, Bridenbaugh PO eds., *Neural blockade in clinical anesthesia and management of pain*. Philadelphia: Lippincott-Raven, 1998:244.

14  Cook TM. Combined spinal-epidural techniques. *Anaesthesia* 2000;**55**:42–64.

15  Giaufre E. Singe shot caudal block. In: Saint-Maurice C, Schulte Steinberg O, eds. *Regional anaesthesia in children*. Fribourg: Mediglobe SA, 1990:81–7.

16  De Leon-Casasola OA, Lema MJ. Postoperative epidural opioid analgesia: what are the choices? *Anesth Analg* 1996;**83**:867–75.

17  Finucane BT. *Complications of regional anesthesia*. New York: Churchill Livingstone, 1999.

18  Halpern S, Preston R. Postdural puncture headache and spinal needle design. *Anesthesiology* 1994;**81**:2376–83.

19  Bier A. Versuche über Cocainisierung des Rückenmarkes. *Deut Zeitschr Chir* 1899;**51**:361–8.

20  Denny NM, Selander DE. Continuous spinal anaesthesia. *Br J Anaesth* 1998;**81**:590–7.

# 4: Intravenous regional anaesthesia

MIKKO T PITKÄNEN

Over 90 years ago a German surgeon, Professor August Bier, introduced an anaesthesia method which is nowadays called intravenous regional anaesthesia (IVRA) or Bier's block.[1] It has gone through relatively small modifications since the beginning of the century and still remains an excellent method for short-lasting day care surgery of the hand and arm.

The overall safety of the method has been documented in several reports. For instance, in an extensive review of regional anaesthesia complications in France the only major complications which Dr Auroy and co-workers[2] reported were three patients with seizures after 11 229 intravenous regional anaesthesia procedures. Another survey from the UK[3] comprised about 45 000 intravenous regional anaesthesia procedures with prilocaine without convulsion, arrhythmia or fatality. The method is also reliable and a success rate of 98.6% without complications was reported in the ambulatory setting for carpal tunnel, carpal ganglion, and trigger finger operations in 732 patients.[4] IVRA is also a useful technique from the economic point of view. The cost of anaesthesia and recovery using IVRA for outpatient hand surgery was reported to be about half of that for general anaesthesia.[5]

The method has certain limitations and is suitable only for short-lasting surgery (<1 hour). Anaesthesia could, in fact, last as long as the tourniquet is inflated but the inflated tourniquet cuff starts to cause pain. This tourniquet pain is a major problem with IVRA as a tourniquet must be used all the time, including during closure of the wound. Even though the method seems relatively simple certain precautions are necessary because the consequences of technical failure may be serious. In the 1980s seven deaths after IVRA were reported.[6] Common to these was that bupivacaine was used and the attending physician was not an anaesthetist. Also, a report of a lost arm, probably due to erroneous injection of a foreign substance, has been published.[7]

IVRA is best suited for arm and hand surgery but can also be used for foot surgery.[8] However, surgery of the whole leg, with a tourniquet around the thigh, is not practical because of the large dose (volume) of local anaesthetic required.

## Technique

Premedication is useful in the ambulatory setting. Either oral diazepam 45–60 min earlier or a small dose of intravenous diazepam just before performing the block can be used. The operation room must be adequately equipped for the treatment of complications. Oxygen, suction, and a ventilation bag with valves, masks and intubation tubes must be available. The patient must be properly monitored; electrocardiogram, blood pressure monitor, and pulse oximeter should be used. The signs of toxicity from local anaesthetics must be monitored, especially during injection, switching the tourniquet cuffs, and deflating the tourniquet. For treatment of complications a rapidly acting hypnotic drug (propofol, thiopentone), short-acting muscle relaxant, vasopressor, anticholinergic agent, and resuscitative medication must be available. The person performing the block must be capable of using the resuscitative apparatus and medication. An IV cannula must always be inserted in the opposite arm.

For injecting the local anaesthetic another IV cannula is inserted on the hand or arm to be operated upon, usually as peripherally as possible, on the dorsum of the hand. It should not be larger than 1.0 mm in diameter. The local anaesthetic must be injected slowly and the small diameter of the cannula prevents overrapid injection. A more proximal vein sometimes has to be used, due to trauma or other reasons. The closer to the tourniquet cuff the local anaesthetic is injected, the more care needs to be taken to avoid high intravenous pressure peaks (see below). The onset of the block after injection into an antecubital vein is markedly slower.[9]

To establish a bloodless arm, a pneumatic tourniquet on the upper arm is needed. The arm must be well padded to protect the skin. The scrubbing of

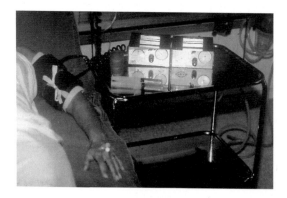

Figure 4.1    Equipment needed for intravenous regional anaesthesia (photo Jukka Alstela)

---

## Box 4.1    Equipment needed for IVRA

- Monitoring: ECG, blood pressure, $SpO_2$
- Resuscitation equipment: $O_2$, suction, positive pressure ventilation, defibrillator available
- Resuscitation medicine and thiopentone or propofol, short-acting muscle relaxant
- IV cannula in the opposite arm
- Double-cuff tourniquet or two separate cuffs
- Checked manometers and pressure devices
- Soft padding under the tourniquet
- Martin's rubber bandage (Esmarch bandage)
- IV cannula (1.0 mm)
- Syringes
- Saline
- Local anaesthetic (prilocaine 5 mg/ml without additives)
- Diazepam, fentanyl, non-steroidal antiinflammatory drug (IV formulation)

---

the operation field must be done carefully to avoid disinfectant getting under the tourniquet. Compression and ischaemia of the skin by the cuff and disinfectant can easily damage the skin. On the upper arm two separate tourniquet cuffs with accurate gauges and manometers should be used. The cuffs must be equipped with straps and security cords which are thoroughly tied around both cuffs. There may not always be space for two separate cuffs and specially designed IVRA double-cuff tourniquets – two cuffs attached to each other – are available. Two cuffs are needed since the second one can be used as a security if the other one accidentally breaks. Switching the pressure from the proximal tourniquet cuff to the distal one can also diminish tourniquet pain.

There is usually some degree of anaesthesia under the distal cuff since it is within the bloodless field where the local anaesthetic primarily distributes. Changing the site of the pressure clearly changes the sensation of tourniquet pain which will provide more time to finish the surgery. If the distal tourniquet starts to become painful, the pressure can be switched back to the proximal tourniquet which may ease the pain to some extent.

The gauges and manometers must be checked at regular intervals. The accuracy of the readings is important: too high a pressure can cause damage to muscles and nerves under the tourniquet while too low a pressure causes leakage of blood to the extremity and also may cause leakage of the local anaesthetic out into the circulation.

The extremity is exsanguinated, usually using a modified von Esmarch bandage often called the Martin bandage. The 10–12 cm wide rubber bandage is wound from the periphery towards the tourniquet cuff. It creates pressure which exceeds the arterial pressure and the vessels of the extremity will be emptied. The bandage is applied over the distal tourniquet cuff and then the cuffs are inflated, first the distal cuff and then the proximal one. The next step is to deflate the distal cuff and remove the Martin bandage. The pressure in the cuff is usually kept 80–100 mmHg higher than the systolic arterial blood pressure. When pressurising the cuffs, the cessation of the pulse should be checked or a pulse oximeter probe used on the affected finger to ascertain the interruption of the circulation. Another way to provide a bloodless field is for the arm to be elevated and at the same time the brachial artery compressed in the axilla. After 2–4 minutes the cuffs can be inflated. This method can be used if the application of the rubber bandage is too painful, for instance because of a fracture.

Before injecting the anaesthetic the arm must be inspected again. If the veins become distended in spite of the inflated tourniquet cuff, the cuff must be deflated and the bandage reapplied. The cuff pressure should now be about 50 mmHg higher. If there is still leakage of blood under the tourniquet, IVRA is not a feasible technique.

Sometimes oozing of blood at the site of surgery is a problem. This is believed to be due to the combined effect of a large volume of local anaesthetics together with continuing blood flow through intramedullary vessels of the bone into the vasculature of the arm. This problem can be diminished with a method called "reIVRA".[10] In a study where the limb was reexsanguinated just before the operation, 15–20 min after injection of the anaesthetic, reIVRA provided a significantly better surgical field without affecting sensory and motor block and actually improved tolerance to the tourniquet pressure. The original Bier's method was to use two bandages, one above the level of operation and another below. The local anaesthetic, procaine 2.5–5.0 mg/ml, volume up to 100 ml, was injected into a vein between these bandages.

When IVRA is used for foot surgery, the tourniquet cuff is placed well below the knee. The upper edge of the tourniquet must be at least 4–5 cm below the head of the fibula as the peroneal nerve is superficially situated and prone to damage. There is no space for two cuffs in this area and the other cuff can be placed on the thigh. It is used only for security reasons and is left deflated. There may be more problems with the tourniquet cuff in IVRA of the lower leg since, in contrast to the upper arm, there are two longitudinal bones and their interspace is not compressed. Leakage of blood or local anaesthetic under the cuff is more probable.

The local anaesthetic is injected slowly, at a rate of approximately

20 ml/min. Even at this speed and injection into a hand vein, peak pressure in the basilic vein can be almost 100 mmHg.[11] Faster injection increases the pressure in the veins and leakage of the local anaesthetic under the tourniquet is possible. In a volunteer study injection of saline 0.75 ml/kg in 20 seconds caused a maximum peak pressure of 255 mmHg.[12]

The block will be established in 10–15 min. Usually, within 30 min the tourniquet starts to cause some discomfort or pain. Switching the pressure of the tourniquet (see above) will usually allow more time for surgery. However, often the tourniquet pain increases and after 60 min intravenous analgesics are needed to diminish the pain. That is why IVRA should not be used for operations which are expected to last more than one hour. The tourniquet can usually be deflated in one step but if the time the tourniquet has been applied is very short (15–20 min), the deflation should be done in 30 second cycles of deflation and reinflation until it is certain that no toxic symptoms will develop. The wound must be closed and haemostasis achieved before opening the tourniquet. The patient must be closely observed during deflation and must be under supervision for at least 30 min after deflation.

## Mechanism of action

August Bier proposed that the mechanism of anaesthesia is first a direct block of nerve endings near the injection site and later, a profound block of the main nerve trunks. Basically he was correct. Studies performed since have not substantially modified his initial idea. First, the peripheral nerve endings become blocked and when the local anaesthetic spreads into the cubital area, the major nerve trunks become blocked. Raj et al[13] used two or more occluding tourniquets and were able to show that even when a distal flow of contrast medium-local anaesthetic mixture was prevented, anaesthesia developed to the most distal parts of the arm. Also radioisotope studies have shown that the local anaesthetic is mainly retained in the antecubital fossa.[14] On the other hand, when injection sites have been compared, injection into a vein in the dorsum of the hand produces anaesthesia faster than injection into a cubital vein.[14] However, the quality of the final surgical block is similar.

Besides the effect of the local anaesthetics on the nerves, ischaemia and hypoxia also have an anaesthetising effect. Pinprick anaesthesia of the arm will develop in about 20 min if saline instead of local anaesthetic is used for IVRA.[15] However, IVRA without local anaesthetic would not be a suitable clinical technique because the effects of ischaemia and the tourniquet pain become uncomfortable and difficult to bear quite early during the course of the technique.

# Local anaesthetics

All local anaesthetics have been used for IVRA. However, since the local anaesthetic is injected directly into a blood vessel safety is especially important. There is always a possibility that the local anaesthetic will enter the circulating blood unintentionally. There may be technical problems with the tourniquet but also, in spite of proper pressure in the tourniquet cuff, leakage of local anaesthetic has been shown to be possible.[16]

Currently, *prilocaine* seems to be the safest of the amino amide local anaesthetics. It is less cardiotoxic and CNS toxic than two other local anaesthetics with approximately similar anaesthetising properties, i.e. lignocaine and mepivacaine. Prilocaine is widely distributed in the body and rapidly metabolised. Usually it is used as a 5 mg/ml concentration with a volume of 40–50 ml (200–250 mg) for IVRA of the arm in adults. The onset time of IVRA of the arm in adults with 40 ml of prilocaine 5 mg/ml has been reported to be 10–12 min, on average. It has also been used in more concentrated (7.5–20 mg/ml) solutions. The higher concentration shortens the onset time but otherwise the block characteristics do not differ much from the less concentrated solution. The risk of CNS toxicity increases when the higher concentrations are used. If the volume of the local anaesthetic solution is decreased, patchy analgesia may ensue.

After the release of the tourniquet there is a moderate increase in blood methaemoglobin levels[17] but not to a level that is accompanied by cyanosis and hypoxia. Haemoglobin is oxidised to methaemoglobin by a metabolite of prilocaine, o-toluidine. However, in order for the methaemoglobin level to cause significant hypoxaemia, it has been estimated that the total dose of administered prilocaine has to exceed 600 mg in an adult.[18] When lignocaine and prilocaine have been compared in equal doses, the speed of onset and recovery and quality of anaesthesia have been similar. The blood concentrations of lignocaine have been greater than those of prilocaine after tourniquet release[17] (Fig. 4.2) possibly reflecting the above-mentioned rapid distribution and elimination of prilocaine. Also complaints of dizziness and light-headedness have been reported after lignocaine.

*Bupivacaine* as a 2.5 mg/ml concentration has been used for IVRA because it had the ability to produce residual analgesia. The haemostasis could be checked and the wound closed after release of the tourniquet. However, an IV dose of 100 mg of bupivacaine (40 ml) can be dangerous and even fatal. Because of the well-documented cardiotoxic potential of bupivacaine, it is no longer recommended for IVRA.

However, recently the slightly less toxic propyl derivative of the same structural (pipecolyl xylidide) family, *S(–)-ropivacaine* as a 0.2% concentration, was found to produce as good IVRA as 0.5% lignocaine.[19] After the deflation of the tourniquet cuff the residual analgesia (hypoalgesia) in the skin of the arm was longer with ropivacaine.

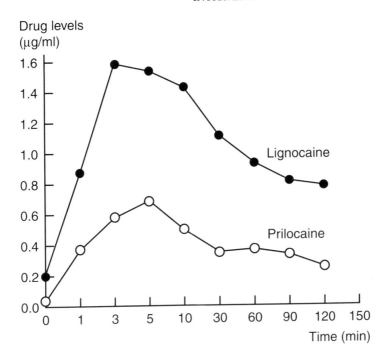

Figure 4.2 Whole-blood lignocaine and prilocaine levels following tourniquet deflation[17]

*Mepivacaine*, another pipecolyl xylidide analogue, has also been used for IVRA but does not offer any benefits over, for example, the less toxic prilocaine.

*2-Chloroprocaine*, an ester-type local anaesthetic which is rapidly metabolised in the bloodstream, would be an almost ideal choice for IVRA. In reports in the 1960s when 2-chloroprocaine was first used for IVRA, thrombophlebitis of the veins in the extremity was reported.[20] A new, additive-free 0.5% 2-chloroprocaine solution seemed to be better tolerated but postinflation irritation of the exposed veins and anaphylactoid skin reactions have been reported.[21,22]

*Articaine* is an amino amide-type local anaesthetic, which has a thiophene ring in its molecule. It has been used mostly in dentistry. In a comparison with prilocaine and lignocaine in IVRA, it was reported to cause much faster onset of anaesthesia.[23] In more recent controlled and blinded studies, however, it has not been possible to repeat these results and there appears to be no difference in blocking action between articaine and prilocaine.[24]

*Pethidine* (meperidine), an opioid with local anaesthetic effects, has also been used for IVRA. It produces a good motor block but pain during the injection and dizziness and nausea after the tourniquet cuff deflation complicate its use.[25]

# Combinations of local anaesthetics and other drugs

Different opioids have been combined with local anaesthetics in order to improve the quality of anaesthesia and the tolerance to tourniquet pain. There are reports on the use of fentanyl (0.1–0.2 mg)[26–28] or morphine (1–6 mg)[29–30] with lignocaine or prilocaine. The anaesthesia benefit has been limited and the higher doses of the opioids have caused dizziness and nausea after deflation of the tourniquet. Pethidine combined with prilocaine, 2.5 mg/ml, in volunteers increased the speed of onset of the block and slowed the recovery.[31] However, again, unpleasant sensations, light-headedness, and nausea as well as temporary swelling of the arm and pruritus occurred when pethidine was used.

When a small dose of a non-depolarising muscle relaxant and fentanyl was combined with a low concentration of local anaesthetic (lignocaine or prilocaine), the quality of anaesthesia was as good as with higher concentrations of the local anaesthetic.[32–34] However, muscle relaxants have caused motor paralysis for several hours after the tourniquet cuff deflation. In volunteers who received mivacurium with prilocaine, the median time to recovery from the motor block was 80 min, the longest recovery time being more than eight hours.[33] Other side effects including diplopia and urticaria were also observed.

Fairly large doses of non-steroidal antiinflammatory drugs (NSAIDs), tenoxicam (20 mg)[35] and ketorolac (60 mg),[36] combined with prilocaine or lignocaine have provided very good postoperative analgesia and also improved the tolerance to tourniquet pain. The effect could not be systemic since the positive effects were observed only if the NSAID was given together with the local anaesthetic into the vasculature of the arm to be anaesthetised. If it was given intravenously to the opposite arm, the beneficial effects were not significant.

Clonidine, an $\alpha_2$-adrenergic agonist, has been added to a local anaesthetic solution in order to improve the quality of the block.[37] It seems to improve the tolerance to tourniquet pain, especially if the tourniquet time is longer than 30 min. Clonidine does not affect the occurrence of postoperative pain to any great extent. The well-known systemic effects of clonidine, hypotension and sedation, have been reported after tourniquet release.

Prilocaine solutions have been alkalinised by adding sodium bicarbonate.[38] This increases the pH and the proportion of the base form of the molecule. The penetration of nerve membranes is thus faster. This prilocaine and sodium bicarbonate mixture has been found to decrease the onset time and improve the quality of anaesthesia.

It is questionable whether any of the proposed or tested mixtures of local anaesthetic and another drug really are of any clinical significance in IVRA. The adequacy of anaesthesia is rarely a problem and many of the additives seem to cause side effects after releasing the tourniquet cuff.

## Additives

When a large volume of local anaesthetic is injected into a vein it is important that no preservatives or antioxidants are included. Erythematous skin reactions in the exposed arm have been observed after the release of the tourniquet when a methylparaben-containing prilocaine solution was used.[39] Naturally, the solutions must not contain adrenaline because of the risk of sustained ischaemia and tissue damage after the tourniquet cuff deflation.

## Indications and contraindications

IVRA is relatively safe and very practical in the ambulatory setting. It is suitable for short-lasting (<1 hour) surgery of the arm or foot when the operation can be finished before deflating the tourniquet. In certain circumstances the surgeon likes to reinstitute the perfusion in the extremity before closing the wound in order to secure perfect haemostasis.

IVRA should not be used in non-cooperative patients, patients with severe hypertensive disease, skeletal muscle disorders or hypersensitivity to local anaesthetics. If there is infection in the area to be anaesthetised, caution must be used.

## Safety

IVRA necessitates injecting a large, potentially toxic amount of local anaesthetic directly into a vein. If there is leakage under the tourniquet, the local anaesthetic in the systemic circulation can cause toxic symptoms. Throughout the block the patient should be awake, or only lightly sedative, and cooperative. During injection he must be frequently asked how he is doing. Even with regularly checked and properly applied tourniquets, leakage of the local anaesthetic under the cuff has been observed.[16] By performing the intravenous injection slowly, pretoxic signs and symptoms (see Chapter 2) can be detected and further injection stopped in time. There should always be a thiopentone or propofol solution nearby for immediate treatment of severe CNS toxicity. As mentioned above, readiness (equipment and drugs) for cardiopulmonary resuscitation is mandatory.

63

1 Bier A. Über einen neuen Weg Localanästhesie an den Gliedmaassen zu erzeugen. *Arch Klin Chir* 1908; **86**:1007–16.
2 Auroy Y, Narchi P, Messiah A *et al.* Serious complications related to regional anesthesia. *Anesthesiology* 1997;**87**:479–86.
3 Bartholomew K, Sloan JP. Prilocaine for Bier's block: how safe is safe? *Arch Emerg Med* 1990; 7:189–95.
4 Dunlop DJ, Graham CM, Waldram MA, Mulligan PJ, Watt JM. The use of Bier's block for day case surgery. *J Hand Surg* (Br) 1995; **20**:679–80.
5 Chilvers CR, Kinahan A, Vaghadia H, Merrick PM. Pharmacoeconomics of intravenous regional anaesthesia vs general anaesthesia for outpatient hand surgery. *Can J Anaesth* 1997;**44**:1152–6.
6 Heath ML. Bupivicaine toxicity and Bier blocks. *Anesthesiology* 1983;**59**:481.
7 Luce EA, Mangubat E. Loss of hand and forearm following Bier block: a case report. *J Hand Surg* (Am) 1983;**8**:280–3.
8 Kim DD, Shuman C, Sadr B. Intravenous regional anesthesia for outpatient foot and ankle surgery: a prospective study. *Orthopedics* 1993;**16**:1109–13.
9 Blyth MJ, Kinninmonth AW, Asante DK. Bier's block: a change of injection site. *J Trauma* 1995;**39**:726–8.
10 Rawal N, Hallén J, Amilon A, Hellstrand P. Improvement in i.v. regional anaesthesia by re-exsanguination before surgery. *Br J Anaesth* 1993;**70**:280–5.
11 Haasio J, Hiippala S, Rosenberg PH. Intravenous regional anaesthesia of the arm. *Anaesthesia* 1989;**44**:19–21.
12 Lawes EG, Johnson T, Pritchard P, Robbins P. Venous pressures during simulated Bier's block. *Anaesthesia* 1984;**39**:147–9.
13 Raj PP, Garcia CE, Burleson JW, Jenkins MT. The site of action of intravenous regional anesthesia. *Anesth Analg* 1972;**51**:776–86.
14 Risdall JE, Young PC, Jones DA, Hett DA. A comparison of intercuff and single cuff techniques of intravenous regional anaesthesia using 0.5% prilocaine mixed with technetium 99m-labelled BRIDA. *Anaesthesia* 1997;**52**:842–8.
15 Rosenberg PH, Heavner JE. Multiple and complementary mechanisms produce analgesia during intravenous regional anesthesia. *Anesthesiology* 1984;**61**:507–10.
16 Rosenberg PH, Kalso EA, Tuominen MK, Linden H. Acute bupivacaine toxicity as a result of venous leakage under the tourniquet cuff during a Bier block. *Anesthesiology* 1983;**58**:95–8.
17 Bader AM, Concepcion M, Hurley RJ, Arthur GR. Comparison of lidocaine and prilocaine for intravenous regional anesthesia. *Anesthesiology* 1988;**69**:409–12.
18 Hjelm M, Holmdahl MH. Clinical chemistry of prilocaine and clinical evaluation of methaemoglobinaemia induced by this agent. *Acta Anaesthesiol Scand* 1965;**16(Suppl)**:161–70.
19 Hartmannsgruber MWB, Silverman DG, Halaszynski TM *et al.* Comparison of ropivacaine 0.2% and lidocaine 0.5% for intravenous regional anesthesia in volunteers. *Anesth Analg* 1999;**89**:727–31.
20 Harris WH. Choice of anesthetic agents for intravenous regional anaesthesia. *Acta Anaesthesiol Scand* 1969; **36(Suppl)**:47–52.
21 Pitkänen M, Suzuki N, Rosenberg PH. Intravenous regional anaesthesia with 0.5% prilocaine or 0.5% chloroprocaine. A double-blind comparison in volunteers. *Anaesthesia* 1992; **47**:618–19.
22 Pitkänen M, Kyttä J, Rosenberg PH. Comparison of 2-chloroprocaine and prilocaine for intravenous regional anaesthesia of the arm: a clinical study. *Anaesthesia* 1993; **48**:1091–3.

23 Simon MAM, Gielen MJM, Alberink N, Vree TB, van Egmond J. Intravenous regional anesthesia with 0.5% articaine, 0.5% lidocaine, or 0.5% prilocaine. *Reg Anesth* 1997;**22**:29–34.

24 Pitkänen MT, Xu M, Haasio J, Rosenberg PH. Comparison of 0.5% articaine and 0.5% prilocaine in intravenous regional anesthesia of the arm: a cross-over study in volunteers. *Reg Anesth Pain Med* 1999;**24**:131–5.

25 Acalovschi I, Cristea T. Intravenous regional anesthesia with meperidine. *Anesth Analg* 1995; **81**:539–43.

26 Armstrong P, Power I, Wildsmith JA. Addition of fentanyl to prilocaine for intravenous regional anaesthesia. *Anaesthesia* 1991; **46**:278–80.

27 Arthur JM, Heavner JE, Mian T *et al.* Fentanyl and lidocaine versus lidocaine for Bier block. *Reg Anesth* 1992; **17**:223–7.

28 Pitkänen MT, Rosenberg PH, Pere PJ, Tuominen MK, Seppälä TA. Fentanyl-prilocaine mixture for intravenous regional anaesthesia in patients undergoing surgery. *Anaesthesia* 1992; **47**:395–8.

29 Gupta A, Björnsson A, Sjöberg F, Bengtsson M. Lack of peripheral analgesic effect of low-dose morphine during intravenous regional anesthesia. *Reg Anesth* 1993; **18**:250–3.

30 Erciyes N, Akturk G, Solak M *et al.* Morphine/prilocaine combination for intravenous regional anesthesia. *Acta Anaesthesiol Scand* 1995; **39**:845–6.

31 Armstrong PJ, Morton CPJ, Nimmo AF. Pethidine has a local anaesthetic action on peripheral nerves in vivo. *Anaesthesia* 1993; **48**:382–6.

32 Abdulla WY, Fadhil NM. A new approach to intravenous regional anesthesia. *Anesth Analg* 1992; **75**:597–601.

33 Elhakim M, Sadek RA. Addition of atracurium to lidocaine for intravenous regional anaesthesia. *Acta Anaesthesiol Scand* 1994; **38**:542–4.

34 Torrance JM, Lewer BMF, Galletly DC. Low-dose mivacurium supplementation of prilocaine i.v. regional anaesthesia. *Br J Anaesth* 1997; **78**:222–3.

35 Jones NC, Pugh SC. The addition of tenoxicam to prilocaine for intravenous regional anaesthesia. *Anaesthesia* 1996; **51**:446–8.

36 Reuben SS, Steinberg RB, Kreitzer JM, Duprat KM. Intravenous regional anesthesia using lidocaine and ketorolac. *Anesth Analg* 1995; **81**:110–13.

37 Gentili M, Bernard J-M, Bonnet F. Adding clonidine to lidocaine for intravenous regional anesthesia prevents tourniquet pain. *Anesth Analg* 1999;**88**:1327–30.

38 Solak M, Akturk G, Erciyes N *et al.* The addition of sodium bicarbonate to prilocaine solution during i.v. regional anesthesia. *Acta Anaesthesiol Scand* 1991;**35**:572–4.

39 Kajimoto Y, Rosenberg ME, Kyttä J *et al.* Anaphylactoid skin reactions after intravenous regional anaesthesia using 0.5% prilocaine with or without preservative – a double-blind study. *Acta Anaesthesiol Scand* 1995;**39**:782–4.

# 5: Modern technical aspects of regional anaesthesia

MICHAEL MÖLLMANN

## Spinal needles

### Needle size and tip configuration

The first human study on spinal anaesthesia, using cocaine, was published by August Bier in 1899.[1] In the initial experiments which the investigators performed on each other, Bier himself developed an intense headache after having lost a substantial amount of cerebrospinal fluid (CSF) via the relatively large puncture needle. He postulated that transdural loss of CSF after spinal puncture could be the cause. This postulation is as valid today as it was 100 years ago and although the daily rate of CSF production far exceeds the conjectural loss of CSF into the peridural compartment after puncture with modern thin needles, this small amount seems to be sufficient to influence the sensitive equilibrium between CSF production and reabsorption over days.

Besides CSF loss, which appears to depend on the needle size and tip configuration, the incidence of postdural puncture headache (PDPH)[2-4] also depends on biometric data, such as age and gender. The risk of PDPH has been found to be increased in young as well as in female patients.

At the end of the 19th century, the needles used for lumbar puncture by Quincke (1891) and Bier (1898) were about twice as large as needles currently used nowadays.[5] Although the relationship between spinal needle size and PDPH was suspected, it took almost 50 years until markedly thinner needles were produced.

Between the 1940s and 1970s, needles of 26 G, 27 G, and even 32 G[6] were tested. Reusable spinal needles, in the early stages made of gold, platinum or nickel, were the standard. After use the needles were flushed with water followed by ether and then autoclaved. This method was not ideal because the tip was commonly "burred" or damaged, leading to more trauma of the dura and soon, the possibility of infection and medicolegal problems was highlighted.

66

The use of very fine gauge needles (29–32 G) by skilled anaesthesiologists led to low PDPH rates but they were more difficult to handle under routine conditions and thus considered "impractical" in clinical use.[8]

As fine gauge needles are associated with a higher rate of technical difficulties and thicker needles with PDPH, a practical compromise has been reached in the use of 25 G to 27 G needles which have become the routine needle sizes in clinical practice in the last 15 years. With the use of 27 G non-cutting pencil-point spinal needles, the incidence of PDPH is around 1%.

In general, spinal needles of two types have been devised: those with a cutting tip and those with a non-cutting tip. The cutting type is represented by the Quincke needle with sharp point and medium length cutting bevel (Fig. 5.1). The Quincke needle (also called the Quincke–Babcock needle) is the standard single-use needle with a sharp tip which carries the theoretical risk of piercing the cauda equina. The sharp point of the needle is quite vulnerable and in clinical conditions up to 15% of the tips have been found to become bent when they encounter bone.[7]

In order to improve puncturing characteristics, a 26 G needle with a two-zone cutting tip has recently been developed[8] (Fig. 5.2). The dural cut made by the tip is smaller than the outside diameter. In vitro, electron microscopy has shown only minimal traumatisation of the dura and a lower rate of CSF leakage compared with a 26 G Quincke-type or a 24 G Sprotte needle.[4] However, the cutting tip of this needle may easily bend when it meets bone during puncture.[9]

The two main designs of the non-cutting (pencil-point) spinal needle are the Whitacre type and the Sprotte type. The original versions of both have been modified through the years.[10,11] The Whitacre needle originally had a more conical and truly pencil-point like tip, whereas the Sprotte needle has a pencil-point tip shaped more like a bullet (Fig. 5.3).

Pencil-point spinal needles are thought to spread rather than sever dural fibres and therefore there should only be minor leakage of CSF through the puncture hole. In fact, the incidence of PDPH has been found to be lower after punctures with pencil-point needles in comparison with cutting-point needles of the same size.[12] As expected, this metaanalysis also showed that an increase in the size of the same needle type resulted in increased incidence of PDPH. Summarising the influence of tip design and needle size together, it could be shown that the incidence of PDPH would be

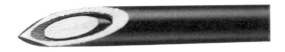

Fig 5.1    A "Quincke" spinal needle

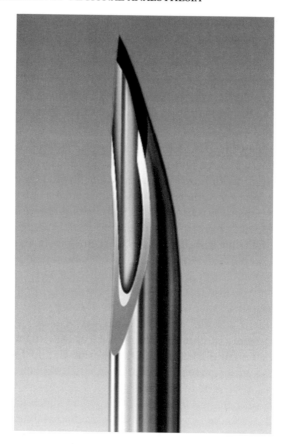

Fig 5.2    A 26 G spinal needle with a two-zone cutting tip

approximately equal when a cutting-point needle or a two gauges larger pencil-point needle is used.

Both the Whitacre and Sprotte needles have a lateral hole on the tip. Originally, Sprotte produced a pencil-point needle which had a longer and wider side hole than the Whitacre design. In clinical practice, this hole allowed the local anaesthetic to escape not only into the spinal but also into the subdural or the epidural space during the injection, which resulted in incomplete anaesthesia.[14] Taking this into consideration, the improved

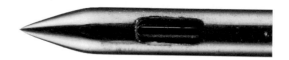

Fig 5.3    Pencil-point spinal needle

version of the Sprotte needle now presents a much smaller orifice which is approximately the same size as that on the modern Whitacre-type needle.

Compared with cutting needles, the tips of non-cutting pencil-point needles are more resistant to mechanical damages. Furthermore, they perforate the dura with a distinct "click" (i.e. a sequence of a gradual increase in resistance when the dura is pushed away by the needle tip followed by a sudden loss of resistance when the tip pierces the dura) which confirms the correct placement of the needle tip. Therefore, both the Whitacre and the Sprotte pencil-point (non-cutting) spinal needles provide safety and reliability under clinical conditions.

In order to improve the CSF backflow through the needle, a 25 G non-cutting Sprotte-type needle (Braun AG, Melsungen, Germany) has recently been tested.[13] Its main advantage is a larger inner diameter (0.32 mm) and therefore better flow characteristics as compared with other 25 G needles. The first clinical trial in 1193 patients showed a failure rate of 1.9% and a PDPH incidence of 1.3%.[13]

## Spinal catheters

Continuous spinal anaesthesia (CSA) is almost as old as spinal anaes-thesia. In 1907, Dean performed the first continuous spinal anaesthesia by leaving the spinal needle in place during the operation.[15] Tuohy was the first to use an intrathecal catheter, i.e. a no. 4 ureteral catheter inserted through a 15 G needle.[16]

Until the late 1980s the use of CSA was limited to poor-risk patients scheduled for lower abdominal or extremity surgery of uncertain duration or morbidly obese parturients undergoing caesarean delivery. Standard epidural equipment was previously used for CSA and is still in use in some centres. Because of a relatively high rate of postdural puncture headache, approximately 10% in elderly patients[17] and even as high as 50% in cae-sarean delivery patients,[18] continuous spinal anaesthesia lost its popularity. At the end of the 1980s, Hurley and Lambert[19] introduced microcatheters (32 G) in an effort to reduce the frequency of spinal headache associated with continuous spinal anaesthesia and interest in its clinical use grew again. However, soon thereafter Riegler et al[20] reported four cases of cauda equina syndrome after continuous spinal anaesthesia performed with hyperbaric local anaesthetic through a microcatheter. As a result of these and other cases of cauda equina syndrome, and in spite of the fact that it was not the catheter but the local anaesthetic solution that was responsible for the com-plications, the Food and Drug Administration (FDA) issued a safety alert in 1992 and banned spinal microcatheters (27 G or thinner) intended for use in continuous spinal anaesthesia from the US market.

Nevertheless, in Europe 26 G and also 28 G polyurethane and polyamide microcatheters are still used for continuous spinal anaesthesia and no reports of cauda equina syndromes have been published. Today, spinal catheters are available from 20 G to 32 G (Table 5.1); these catheters can be introduced by needles 18 G up to 27 G.

*Table 5.1   Continuous spinal catheter types*

| Type | Material | Gauge | Needle |
|---|---|---|---|
| Epidural | Nylon, Teflon | 19, 20 | 16–18 |
| Epidural | Polyamide | 20 | 18 |
| Paediatric epidural | Polyurethane | 24 | 20 |
| Spinal | Nylon | 24, 28 | 20, 22 |
| Spinal (catheter over the needle)* | Nylon | 22, 24 | 27, 29 |
| Spinal | Nylon | 27 | 22, 25, 26 |
| Spinal | Polyamide | 28, 32 | 22 |

* An epidural Crawford-type needle is used as introducer

In response to the practical limitations of microcatheters and restrictions on their use, the latest development in continuous spinal anaesthesia has been the catheter-over-the-needle system that consists of either a 22 G catheter introduced over a 27 G spinal needle (Quincke type) or a 24 G catheter introduced over a 29 G spinal needle, with the tip of the needle protruding a few millimetres outside the catheter (Fig. 5.4) (Spinocath™, Braun AG, Melsungen, Germany).[21] The catheter-over-the-needle design eliminates the leakage of CSF because the catheter seals the dural puncture hole immediately. The macrocatheter size allows for a high flow rate providing a good mixture and dilution of the anaesthetic agent with CSF by easy barbotage and is therefore thought to reduce the risk of cauda equina syndrome. The 27 G (29 G) spinal needle inside the catheter is longer than

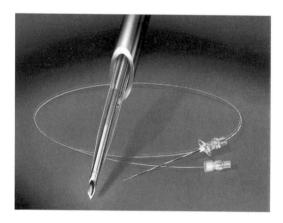

Fig 5.4   A catheter-over-the-needle continuous spinal anaesthesia system

the epidural introducer needle. This needle has a proximal side hole for fast CSF backflow into the catheter and CSF can easily be detected. The spinal needle is connected to a pullwire which extends beyond the proximal end of the catheter and allows the spinal needle to be pulled out of the catheter after intrathecal placement.

For the placement of the catheter, a special straight epidural introducer needle is offered because a standard Tuohy needle with the curved Huber tip would bend the catheter. The resultant friction between the needle and the catheter would not allow the typical distinct perception of the penetration of dura mater. The introducer in this catheter-over-the-needle system is a Crawford-type epidural needle which has the same bevel grind as a Tuohy needle with similar puncturing characteristics. When this epidural needle is placed into the lumbar epidural space, the spinal needle, which is covered by the catheter, is advanced through the needle into the subarachnoid space. When the puncture is successful, the backflow of CSF into the catheter should be seen in a few seconds. Then the catheter is advanced 2–4 cm over the spinal needle, which should be held immobilised and subsequently pulled out with the attached thin metal pullwire. This system guarantees that the catheter fills the entire hole in the dura and thus prevents leakage of CSF that could result in PDPH. Because of the short distance of catheter insertion, the tip should always be at the level of the puncture.[17,22]

In a prospective multicentre study, 247 patients (age 18–93 years) undergoing elective surgery and/or pain therapy were given CSA using the catheter-over-the-needle system(22 G/27 G). In 75.3%, the advancement of the spinal catheter and the aspiration of CSF were regarded as "easy"; in 1.2%, aspiration of CSF was not possible. Within two seconds, appearance of CSF could be observed in 48.2% of the patients. In two recent reports the catheter-over-the-needle technique was found to be at least as good as conventional microcatheter techniques for CSA when used by anaesthesiologists with great experience of CSA.[22,23]

## Epidural needles and catheters

Most clinicians exclusively employ single-use epidural needles such as the curved-tip Tuohy-type needle (Fig. 3.8, p. 48). The Crawford and Hustead designs are less popular.

Since the development of the Tuohy needle more than 50 years ago, no significant changes in needle design have taken place. Therefore, only two new systems will be presented below: the "flexible-tip" epidural catheter system and the "Mancao needle".

When performing epidural anaesthesia, unintentional puncture of the dura mater remains a risk, especially for the novice anaesthetist. In the "flexible-tip" catheter system there is either a metallic spring-wire tip or a flexible distal portion of the catheter that should prevent intravasal placement, reduce the rate of paraesthesia, and prevent unintentional dural perforation. These catheters are quite expensive and are generally used only for special indications (e.g. chronic pain). Limited experience indicates that the incidence of paraesthesia caused by the puncture when such a "flexible-tip" catheter is used is lower than with the use of ordinary "stiff" catheters.

The other principle consists of an epidural two-cannula system, the so-called "Mancao needle", which has a bevelled tip that should improve puncture quality. When the tip is in place in front of the ligamentum flavum, the stylet is removed and replaced by the cannula. The rounded tip of this inner cannula should guarantee that a puncture of the dura mater is unlikely. Furthermore, a blunt and rounded opening allows easy positioning of the catheter in the epidural space and by correct fixation of the inner cannula withdrawal of the catheter is possible. The needle may then be rotated 360° whereby the epidural catheter can be directed either cephalad or caudad. Theoretically, this system looks promising and might make the placing of the epidural needle easier and unintentional puncture of the dura mater almost impossible. This would result in increased safety of this commonly performed regional anaesthetic technique.

Despite years of use, there is still no practical way to confirm correct epidural catheter placement. Tsui et al[24] therefore used electrical stimulation, with a positive motor response to stimulation interpreted as an indication that the catheter is in the epidural space and a negative response interpreted as incorrect catheter positioning. This might be an alternative to the current test dose, i.e. 3 ml 1.5% lignocaine with 1:200 000 adrenaline, used to minimise the possibility of accidental intravascular and subarachnoid catheter placement. Younger anaesthetists in the beginning of their training in particular could gain from this electrical stimulation method.

When performing regional blocks in children, epidural, spinal or caudal, there are some risks of developing latent epidermoid tumors because of the use of non-styleted needles. Thus it is recommended that a stylet should always be used, not only in spinal but also in caudal blocks.[25]

Special paediatric needles such as paediatric epidural, single-shot epidural, spinal, and caudal needles in different sizes and lengths are available. However, for practical manipulatory purposes, the sizes of the paediatric needles cannot be directly proportional to that of the patient and, therefore, epidural and spinal blocks in children are often performed with similar sized needles as in adults. In order to detect signs and symptoms of nerve contact before permanent damage might occur, in children epidural and spinal blocks should be performed as a rule only in awake or lightly sedated patients.

# Combined spinal and epidural anaesthesia

The first combined spinal and epidural (CSE) technique was described in 1937.[26] Using a single needle, Soresi injected local anaesthetic into the epidural space before advancing and performing a subarachnoid injection.

In the 1970s and 1980s, before the development of special CSE sets, a double-segment CSE technique (epidural catheter and spinal needle in different interspaces) was practised in obstetric anaesthesia.[27] The single-segment or so-called "needle-through-needle" technique introduced in 1982 by Coates[28] and Mumtaz et al[29] has attained great popularity. This technique allows the extradural needle to guide the spinal needle in the midline into the depths of the dura mater and only a single puncture is required.

The single-segment technique with epidural catheter placement following the spinal injection has undergone several technical modifications. It may be the current method of choice in most departments but some problems still remain.

## The risk of intrathecal catheter placement

The risk of epidural catheter migration through the hole in the dura made by the spinal needle is especially high if multiple punctures have been necessary; this intrathecal catheter placement might result in total spinal anaesthesia and increase the risk of PDPH. In order to reduce the risk of intrathecal migration of the catheter, the Tuohy needle orifice may be redirected by turning 180° after the dural puncture with the spinal needle but this manoeuvre is not risk free as it may bore a hole in the dura.

Epidural needles for CSE with a hole or "back-eye" punched in the curved tip were first described by Hanaoka in 1986.[30] This needle has an additional aperture near the main distal orifice, which allows the spinal needle to follow a straight course. In some CSE sets a plastic centring sleeve covers the shaft of the spinal needle, except near its tip. This centres the spinal needle in the epidural needle lumen and ensures that it will pass through the back-eye[31]. In another modification, the spinal needle reaches the dura without contacting the epidural catheter. In addition, an adequate distance between epidural catheter and dura mater is ensured which prevents the catheter from reaching the intrathecal zone. With the use of such combinations the risk of intrathecal catheter placement can be considered only theoretical (Fig. 5.5).[32]

## The epidural test and/or top-up dose

The epidural catheter can be used after surgery when the block wears off and pain starts to appear. Then the situation may be a little more

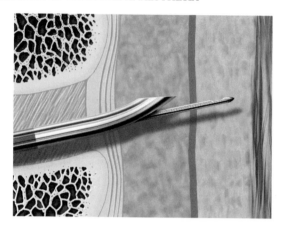

Fig 5.5 A CSE epidural needle with a "back-eye" and a centring sleeve on the shaft of the spinal needle

problematic than when the catheter is required to adjust the initial spinal block or to prolong the duration of anaesthesia. The correct interpretation of the catheter tip position may be difficult because of the partial block already present. At this moment, i.e. just after the end of surgery, even the injection of pure saline may increase the level of spinal block or deepen the partial block. A small dose of plain lignocaine (e.g. 30 mg) has been suggested which should increase the level of the present block by no more than two segments.

The performance of CSE by the double-segment technique or with double-lumen needles allows testing of the correct position of the catheter before the initial induction of the spinal block. However, in any case, the possibility of catheter migration at a later stage should always be kept in mind.

## Metallic particles

At the beginning of the use of the needle-through-needle technique, up to the early 1990s, there was much concern about fine metal particles abraded by the spinal needle from the inner ground edge of the Tuohy needle possibly being introduced into the patient when performing CSE. Back-eye needles were supposed to reduce scratching. Latterly, however, this discussion has faded since it has not been possible to find clinically detectable sequelae that would have indicated a causal relationship.[33,34]

74

## Technical difficulties

In early reports of the needle-through-needle technique the spinal anaesthesia failure rate was 10–25%.[35] Of practical concern was the impossibility of obtaining cerebrospinal fluid, which might indicate a deviation from the midline. Another reason was the limited protrusion distance of the spinal needle from the tip of the epidural needle. Most measured protrusion distances were between 10 and 12 mm, which might not be enough to reach the subarachnoid space and the CSF in about 10% of adult patients.

Therefore, longer spinal needles were required. Some of the technical difficulties encountered with these have been solved by locking the spinal needle after entering the subarachnoid space. One practical modification, called the "docking device", is placed onto the proximal opening of the Tuohy needle and the spinal needle is advanced through it. When the tip of the spinal needle has reached the subarachnoid space, clockwise turning of the device locks the spinal needle in its position (Fig. 5.6). Another locking system involves a spinal needle with a "press-down knob" and when this is pressed it allows the introduction of the spinal needle through the epidural needle. When the dural perforation is felt and CSF backflow is verified, the knob is released and the spinal needle will be locked in this position and no further manipulation is necessary.

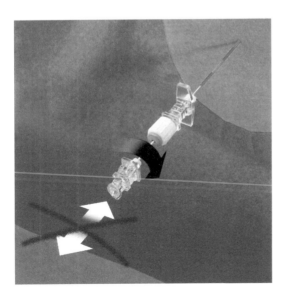

Fig 5.6    A CSE "docking device"

## Neurological problems and sequelae

The possible risk of dural tap is still subject to debate but large series could show that this risk is lower than with intended epidural anaesthesia. In addition, postoperative backache has been the reason for some anaesthetists to give up CSE but may depend on technical skills and the equipment used. Neither cauda equina syndrome nor transient neurological symptoms (TNSs) have been described more frequently after CSE than after pure spinal techniques. Use of the "docking" or locking needle CSE sets seems to be associated with a low incidence of paraesthesia and therefore they might increase the safety of CSE.

# Plexus blocks and nerve stimulators

Blockade of the brachial plexus with local anaesthetics can provide anaesthesia for the upper extremity, from the shoulder to the fingertips. All nerves of the brachial plexus are surrounded by a fascial sheath (complete or partial) which forms an elongated tubular compartment. When performing a (brachial) plexus block, the most striking point is the question of how to identify the correct plexus structures. There are several methods that have yielded high success rates, especially eliciting a paraesthesia with the needle point, using a nerve stimulator or recognising the "click" as the needle enters the sheath.

There are sets available for plexus anaesthesia that consist of an immobile needle for "single-shot" techniques without nerve stimulation but with the need to elicite paraesthesia. These combinations offer a short-bevelled needle with an outer diameter of 24 G which allows the identification of the perivascular space by the distinct "click" felt on piercing the perivascular sheath and reduces the possibility of nerve damage. This needle is connected with a flexible extension tubing which allows the needle to be held firmly within the perivascular space while the syringe is being attached to the hub and injection performed – the "immobile needle technique".

The practice of eliciting paraesthesia (touching the nerve with the needle tip) in order to identify the correct nerve structures has become a subject of discussion.[36,37] Animal experiments and clinical observations suggest that the use of sharp needles might lead to peripheral nerve injury[38] but opposite views have also been presented.[39]

Nerve stimulator techniques for peripheral nerve blocks have been developed.[40,41] These systems, which are the main technical development in plexus block techniques in the last decade, should allow a smooth and target-directed procedure to position the needle tip close to the nerve. In addition, it is well tolerated by the patient because it is no longer necessary to elicit paraesthesia.

In modern apparatus selectable stimulus duration offers the choice of stimulating motor fibres of mixed nerves or of stimulating sensory fibres for the location of pure sensory nerves. The nerve stimulator offers switchable linear current ranges of 0–1 mA and 0–5 mA, selectable pulse duration (selective stimulation of motor fibres for 0.1 ms and additional stimulation of sensory fibres at 1.0 mA), acoustic and optical stimulus indication, and various alarm functions. A precise measurement of the stimulus current delivered should allow accurate positioning of the needle tip close to the nerve; the needle has a special coating and features a non-cutting bevel. There is a wide range of different needle types available; the needle acting as a pinpoint electrode concentrates the entire stimulus current at the needle tip and supports precise nerve localisation.

When using a nerve stimulator and insulated block needles to identify neural structures, the cathode terminal of the stimulator should be connected to the stimulating needle. First, the needle has to be introduced into the subcutaneous tissue. Then a peripheral motor response to stimulation is sought by using a moderate current, for example 1 mA. When a clear peripheral motor response is gained, the current output is decreased and, ideally, a motor response should still be elicited with a current of lower than 0.5 mA (even <0.3 mA) without having to touch the nerve with the needle tip.[41] The anaesthetist should be aware of the fact that a current higher than 0.5 mA can stimulate through the sheath and therefore result in a motor response (twitch) without obtaining a motor blockade.

This technique is usually indicated in order to localise mixed nerves for plexus and peripheral nerve blocks by selective stimulation of motor fibres. In addition, pure sensory nerves (for example, lateral cutaneous nerve of thigh) can be located using a longer pulse duration to stimulate sensory fibres, which might be useful for nerve blocks in pain treatment.[42]

Possible indications for continuous plexus blocks are long-duration anaesthesia for prolonged operations on the upper limb, postoperative analgesia,[43] prolonged treatment for painful conditions (complex regional pain syndrome, cancer pain), and pain-free active physiotherapy. Similar to the single-shot technique, there are several catheter sets for continuous plexus blockades with and without nerve stimulation available today. These follow the "over-the-needle design" which means that the diameter of the polyamide or nylon catheter with an atraumatic tip will be smaller than the puncture hole made by the cannula. The introducing cannulas are still rather large (16–18 G), which means some discomfort for the patient and possible leakage of some of the local anaesthetic solution through the hole. Therefore, further improvement in the design of currently available cannula and catheter sets would be desirable.

In the case of a lumbar plexus block ("three-in-one-block"), a block of the three main components, i.e. the femoral nerve, the obturator nerve and the lateral femoral cutaneous nerve, must be achieved. The identification of the femoral nerve with a nerve stimulator is relatively easy but a catheter must be introduced sufficiently far into the femoral nerve sheath to guarantee an adequate block of the other main nerves too.[44] The Seldinger technique, with a flexible-tip introducer (guidewire), is useful for correct catheter placement.[45]

## Patient-controlled analgesia

In recent years, the administration of opioids via patient-controlled analgesia (PCA) systems for the management of postoperative pain has gained increasing popularity. The increasing use of this technique is accompanied by ongoing widespread fear with regard to the safety of such self-administration by the patient. This concern focuses on the incidence of respiratory depression with potentially fatal consequences, the risk of addiction and several other adverse effects such as sedation, nausea, and depression of gastrointestinal function.[46,47]

By avoiding opioids, regional anaesthetic techniques provide excellent analgesia in an alert, cooperative patient untroubled by nausea. Peripheral nerve blocks can provide adequate analgesia over a limited field with minimal systemic effect and have been used satisfactorily as single-shot techniques. Nevertheless, they have not yet gained acceptance for prolonged postoperative analgesia although a catheter can be inserted through the fascial sheaths which surround major neurovascular compartments and the PCA principle could be applied. Although primarily developed for intravenous use, the system has also been successfully applied epidurally (PCEA) using local anaesthetics, for example in obstetric epidural analgesia,[48,49] and local anaesthetics plus opioid in continuous postoperative epidural anaesthesia.[50,51]

Despite the obvious safety of PCA, avoidable instances of respiratory depression still occur with this technique. The causes of such problems, related to the administration of intravenous opioid by PCA apparatus, may be classified as operator errors, patient-related errors, and equipment problems.[52] Operator errors include incorrect programming, accidental bolusing during syringe changes, inappropriate prescription of dose or lockout interval, drug errors, and misconnection or absence of Y-connectors with appropriate antireflux and antisyphon valves. The most common patient-related errors seem to be the use of the pumps by others (especially relatives) and failure to understand the device. These errors can best be avoided by a careful selection of suitable patients. Clear explanations need to be given to patients and relatives regarding the problem of use of the PCA button by someone other than the patient because such abuse breaches the inherent safety of the technique.

Equipment problems are becoming more and more rare because of the development of newer PCA pump systems in the last few years. The very first systems were quite large but parameters such as infusion volume, infusion rate, and lockout interval could be programmed. For a valid demand, the patient had to press the button twice a second, a task only patients with clear consciousness can manage. In some newer designs, an additional basal infusion rate of the analgesic drug could also be programmed.

Later PCA pump systems became smaller and more lightweight (Fig. 5.7). These new systems are portable, so that patients can move about freely, and are powered by batteries with a duration of more than 400 hours. As the use of these PCA pumps is easy for the patient to learn, there is now a version in which a "smart card", with data on drug concentration, bolus doses, lockout intervals, and basal infusion rates, can be inserted into the pump. The special software programmes on these cards support an individual therapy for the patient so a change of the pain management does not require another pump system but can be effected with a new software card. Thus, the patient does not need to learn how to use another system. The system works with an infusion reservoir (from 50 up to 250 ml) that offers the possibility of individual infusion rate management from 0.1 up to 100 ml/h.

Several companies offer elastomeric infusion pumps that are designed to give clinicians and nurses, either in hospital or in the home environment, the option of delivering to the patient predetermined amounts of medication in a continuous manner. The basic principle of these devices is that an elastic membrane, which consists of one or two layers, is connected to an extension tube which contains a flow regulation device, which is then connected to the venous, arterial or spinal access of the patient. Delivery to the patient is maintained by positive pressure from the elastic membrane.

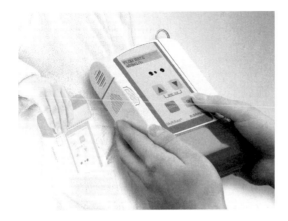

Fig 5.7    A portable PCA pump system

The rate of flow is determined by the combination of the flow regulation device and the positive pressure of the membrane. The pressure of the membrane allows delivery of the solution against the back pressure of catheters and blood pressure in the veins and arteries. Back pressure will affect the flow rate. These elastomeric pumps are independent of mains power supply or batteries so the patient can be ambulatory, secure in the knowledge that the pump will continue to infuse wherever he or she may be.

Concerning postoperative patient-controlled regional analgesia at home, Rawal and co-workers reported a study of patients who underwent a variety of surgical procedures and were supplied with a multihole, thin (22 G) epidural catheter connected to a disposable, elastomeric (balloon) pump containing 50–100 ml bupivacaine 0.125% or 0.25%.[53] A simple procedure of opening and closing a clamp allowed patients to self-administer a prescribed dose of local anaesthetic. When analgesia was no longer required, the patients removed the catheter and discarded the pump. Pain relief was graded good to excellent by 89% of the patients, onset of analgesia was experienced within 5 min, and patient follow-up did not reveal any infection or technical problems.

In general, patient satisfaction with patient-controlled analgesia is extremely high. These high satisfaction scores are most probably best explained by the provision of personal control over delivery of pain relief in a hospital environment and at home. Despite this, systemic administration of opioids via a PCA or local anaesthetic plus opioid in PCEA seems to be associated with a number of patients who experience inadequate analgesia and relevant side effects, in particular nausea, vomiting, and sedation.

1 Bier A. Versuche über die Cocainisierung des Rückenmarkes. *Deut Zeitschr Chir* 1899;**51**:361.

2 Gielen M. Post dural puncture headache (PDPH): a review. *Reg Anesth* 1989:**14**:101–7.

3 Greene HM. Lumbar puncture and the prevention of postpuncture headache. *JAMA* 1926;**86**:391–2.

4 Holst D, Möllmann M, Ebel C, Hausmann R, Wendt M. In vitro investigation of cerebrospinal fluid leakage after dural puncture with various spinal needles. *Anesth Analg* 1998;**87**:1331–5.

5 Brown DL, Fink BR. The history of neural blockade and pain management. In: Cousins JM, Bridenbraugh PO, eds. *Neural blockade in clinical anesthesia and management of pain*. Philadelphia: Lippincott-Raven, 1998:3–27.

6 Frumin MJ. Spinal anesthesia using a 32-gauge needle. *Anesthesiology* 1969;**30**:599–603.

7 Puolakka R, Jokinen M, Pitkänen MT, Rosenberg PH. Comparison of postanaesthetic sequelae after clinical use of 27-gauge cutting and noncutting spinal needles. *Reg Anesth* 1997;**22**:521–6.

8 Scott D, Dittmann M, Clough DGF et al. Atraucan™: a new needle for spinal anaesthesia. *Reg Anesth* 1993;**18**:213–17.

9   Rosenberg PH, Pitkänen MT, Hakala P, Andersson LC. Microscopic analysis of the tips of thin spinal needles after subarachnoid puncture. *Reg Anesth* 1993;**21**:35–40.

10  Hart JR, Whitacre RG. Pencil-point needle in prevention of post spinal hedache. *JAMA* 1951;**147**:657–8.

11  Sprotte G, Schedel R, Pajunk H. Eine "atraumatische" Universalkanüle für einzeitige Regionalanästhesien. *Regional-Anästhesie* 1987;**10**:104–8.

12  Halpern S, Preston R. Postdural puncture headache and spinal needle design. *Anesthesiology* 1994;**81**:1376–83.

13  Möllmann M. Subdurale, intraarachnoidale Ausbreitung von Lokalanästhetika. *Der Anaesthesist* 1992;**41**:685–8.

14  Krommendijk E, Verheijen R, van Dijk B, Spoelder E, Gielen M, de Lange J. The PENCAN 25-gauge needle: a new pencil-point needle for spinal anaesthesia tested in 1,193 patients. *Reg Anesth Pain Med* 1999;**24(1)**:43–50.

15  Dean HP. Discussion on the relative value of inhalational and injection methods of inducing anaesthesia. *BMJ* 1907;**5**:869–77.

16  Tuohy EB. Continuous spinal anaesthesia: its usefulness and technique involved. *Anesthesiology* 1944;**5**:142–8.

17  Pitkänen M. Continuous spinal anaesthesia and analgesia. *Tech Reg Anesth Pain Manag* 1998;**2**:96–102.

18  Norris MD, Leighton BL. Continuous spinal anesthesia after accidental dural puncture in parturients. *Reg Anesth* 1990;**15**:285–7.

19  Hurley RH, Lambert DH. Continuous spinal anaesthesia with a microcatheter technique: the experience in obstetrics and general surgery. *Reg Anesth* 1989;**14**:3–8.

20  Riegler ML, Drasnker K, Krejcie TC *et al.* Cauda equina syndrome after continuous spinal anaesthesia. *Anesth Analg* 1991;**72**:275–81.

21  Möllmann M, van Steenberge A, Sell A *et al.* Spinocath™, a new approach to continuous anaesthesia – preliminary results of a multicenter trial (abstract). *Int Monitor* 1996;**8**:47.

22  DeAndrès J, Valia J, Olivares A, Bellver J. Continuous spinal anesthesia: a comparative study of standard microcatheter and Spinocath. *Reg Anesth Pain Med* 1999;**24(2)**:110–16.

23  Muralidhar V, Kaul HL, Mallick P. Over-the-needle versus microcatheter-through-needle technique for continuous spinal anesthesia: a preliminary study. *Reg Anesth Pain Med* 1999; **24**: 417–21.

24  Tsui B, Gupta S, Finucane B. Determination of epidural catheter placement using nerve stimulation in obstetric patients. *Reg Anesth Pain Med* 1999;**24(1)**:17–23.

25  Broadman LM. Where should advocacy for pediatric patients end and concerns for patient safety begin? (editorial) *Reg Anesth* 1997;**22(3)**:205–8.

26  Soresi AL. Episubdural anaesthesia. *Anesth Analg* 1937;**16**:306–10.

27  Brownridge P. Epidural and subarachnoid analgesia for elective caesarean section. *Anaesthesia* 1981;**36**:70.

28  Coates MB. Combined subarachnoid and epidural techniques: a single space technique for surgery of the hip and lower limb. *Anaesthesia* 1982;**37**:89–90.

29  Mumtaz MH, Daz M, Kuz M. Combined subarachnoid and epidural techniques: another single space technique for orthopaedic surgery. *Anaesthesia* 1982;**37**:90.

30  Hanaoka K. Experience in the use of Hanaoka's needles for spinal-continuous

epidural anaesthesia (500 cases). Seventh Asian-Australian Congress of Anaesthesiologists, Hong Kong, 1986.

31 Joshi GP, McCarroll SM. Combined spinal-epidural anesthesia using needle-through-needle technique. *Anesthesiology* 1993;**78**:406–7.

32 Holmström B, Rawal N. Combined spinal-epidural block: what can we learn from epiduroscopy? *Tech Reg Anesth Pain Manag* 1997;**1**:107–12.

33 Hermann N, Molin J, Knape KG. No additional metal particle formation using the needle through needle combined spinal/epidural technique. *Acta Anaesthesiol Scand* 1996;**40**:227–31.

34 Holst D, Möllmann M, Schymroszcyk B, Ebel C, Wendt M. No risk of metal toxicity in combined spinal-epidural anaesthesia. *Anesth Analg* 1999;**88**:393–7.

35 Cook TM. Combined spinal-epidural techniques (review article). *Anaesthesia* 2000;**55**:42–64.

36 Selander D, Edskage S, Wolff T. Paraesthesia or no paraesthesia. *Acta Anaesthesiol Scand* 1979;**23**:27–33.

37 Finucane BT. Complications of brachial plexus anesthesia. In: Finucane BT, ed. *Complications of regional anesthesia*. New York: Churchill Livingstone, 1999:56–76.

38 Selander D, Dhuner KG, Lundborg G. Peripheral nerve injury due to injection needles used for regional anaesthesia. *Acta Anaesthesiol Scand* 1977;**21**:182–8.

39 Rice ASC, McMahon SB. Peripheral nerve injury caused by injection needles used in regional anaesthesia: influence of bevel configuration studied in a rat model. *Br J Anaesth* 1992;**69**:433–8.

40 Greenblatt GM, Denson JS. Needle nerve stimulator-locator: nerve blocks with a new instrument for locating nerves. *Anesth Analg Curr Res* 1962;**41**:599–602.

41 Pither C. Nerve stimulation. In: Raj PP, ed. *Clinical practice of regional anesthesia*. New York: Churchill Livingstone, 1991:161–9.

42 Shannon J, Lang SA, Yip R, Gerard M. Lateral femoral cutaneous nerve block revisited. A nerve stimulator technique. *Reg Anesth* 1995;**20**:100–4.

43 Tuominen M, Haasio J, Hekali R, Rosenberg PH. Continuous interscalene brachial plexus block: clinical efficacy, technical problems and bupivacaine plasma concentrations. *Acta Anaesthesiol Scand* 1989;**33**:84–8.

44 Postel J, März P. Die kontinuierliche Blockade des Plexus lumbalis ("3-in-1 Block") in der perioperativen Schmerztherapie. *Regional-Anaesthesie* 1984;**7**:140–3.

45 Marhofer P, Schrögendorfer K, Wallner T, Koinig H, Mayer N, Kapral S. Ultrasonographic guidance reduces the amount of local anesthetics for 3-in-1-blocks. *Reg Anesth Pain Med* 1998;**23**:584–8.

46 Looi-Lyons LC, Chung FF, Chan VW, McQuestion M. Respiratory depression: an adverse outcome during patient controlled analgesia therapy. *J Clin Anesth* 1996;**8**:151–6.

47 Lehmann KA. Intravenous patient-controlled analgesia: postoperative pain management and research. In: Chrubasik J, Cousins M, Martin E eds., *Advances in pain therapy II*. Berlin: Springer-Verlag, 1993:65–93.

48 Gambling DR, McMorland GH, Yu P, Laszlo C. Comparison of patient-controlled epidural analgesia and conventional "top-up" injections during labor. *Anesth Analg* 1990;**70**:256–61.

49 Paech MJ. Epidural analgesia in labour. Constant infusion plus patient-controlled boluses. *Anaesth Intens Care* 1991;**19**:32–9.

50 Cooper DW, Turner G. Patient-controlled extradural analgesia to compare

bupivacaine, fentanyl and bupivacaine with fentanyl in the treatment of postoperative pain. *Br J Anaesth* 1993;**70**:503–7.

51 Liu S, Allen H, Olsson G. Patient-controlled epidural analgesia with bupivacaine and fentanyl on hospital wards: prospective evidence with 1,030 surgical patients. *Anesthesiology* 1998;**88**:688–95.

52 Baird M, Schug SA. Safety aspects of postoperative pain relief. *Pain Digest* 1996;**6**:219–25.

53 Rawal N, Hylander J, Nydahl PA, Olofsson I, Gupta A. Survey of postoperative analgesia following ambulatory surgery. *Acta Anaesthesiol Scand* 1997;**41**:1017–22.

# 6: Local anaesthesia in ambulatory surgery

JAN JAKOBSSON

## Inpatient surgery versus outpatient surgery

In recent years the surgical service has changed dramatically. In the past patients remained in hospital for several days after the surgical intervention. Today, an increasing number of procedures are carried out on an outpatient basis and there are many reasons for this trend towards a shift from inhospital service to an ambulatory one.

Cost is without doubt one of the most powerful factors influencing the change in practice. The introduction of less invasive/traumatic surgical techniques, new fast-acting analgesics, and anaesthetics is also of importance. An increasing understanding of the physiological process associated with surgical trauma and its management has had a major impact.[1,2] Regardless of the reasons, it is clear that many medical centres make big efforts to increase the ratio in favour of ambulatory versus inhospital procedures.[3,4] More complex procedures are carried out on the elderly and sicker patients on an outpatient basis.

In view of this, ambulatory anaesthesia is becoming a major part of the anaesthesiologist's workload. The goal is to provide safe and comfortable anaesthesia and fast recovery of mental function with minimum undesirable side effects such as pain, emesis, dizziness, headache, and drowsiness. Many ambulatory patients can be discharged following their surgical procedures into their home environment under appropriate and controlled conditions.

## General anaesthesia versus local/regional anaesthesia

Major morbidity associated with ambulatory anaesthesia is rare.[5] Pain from the incision area, emesis, dizziness, drowsiness, headache, and sore throat are, however, symptoms frequently recalled after general anaesthesia.[3,6] Pain and emesis are, in fact, major indications for non-anticipated readmission of the operated patient.[4,7]

Apart from these distressing symptoms, general anaesthesia is often associated with varying degrees of mental/cognitive impairment that may last for several days.[8] These symptoms may have implications for the postsurgical course. Patients may forget instructions given at discharge and may even be incapable of performing normal daily activities. Although all patients should be provided with written instructions these may not be complete for each individual patient.

Patients operated upon under local or regional anaesthesia will experience about the same degree of postoperative pain after block reversal as general anaesthesia patients. However, they experience less cognitive impairment, emesis, drowsiness, and sore throat postoperatively.[9,10] Receiving information during the procedure may also have a positive impact. Patients undergoing surgery under local or regional anaesthesia are therefore more likely to recall information and instructions given perioperatively.

## Benefits and drawbacks of local anaesthesia

Local anaesthesia is a natural part of office-based minor surgery. Local anaesthesia alone or in combination with other drugs/techniques also has a prominent place in more extensive cases performed in the ambulatory setting. A number of different combinations can be used with local anaesthesia as the basic component (Box 6.1).

The use of local anaesthesia alone or in combination with analgesics, sedation or light general anaesthesia will without doubt increase during the coming years.[11] The features of local anaesthesia make it a logical choice for use in ambulatory surgery. Regional or local anaesthesia affects only part of the body. In particular, it has no effect on brain function provided that toxicity is avoided. The patient is awake and autonomic functions and reflexes of the unblocked part of the body are intact. In the majority of situations there is no pharmacological interference with respiration, circulation, and protective reflexes. These features have great implications both peroperatively and postoperatively, eliminating the entire period of recovery of consciousness. The need for postoperative monitoring of vital functions is reduced. The patients may fulfil criteria to bypass the high-dependency recovery area, facilitating the so-called "fast track" organisation.[12] The patient will also in most instances have good analgesia for several hours postoperatively.

It is important to emphasise that the choice of anaesthetic technique should not be an "either/or" discussion but a question of how the procedure can be managed optimally with as few residual effects, such as pain, nausea, and cognitive impairment, as possible. Many techniques and combinations are possible (Box 6.1), all with the goal of creating a safe and effective intraoperative course with a fast and "pleasant" recovery.

---

**Box 6.1    Possible combinations including local anaesthesia for use in ambulatory surgery.**

Topical anaesthesia
Local anaesthesia
Local anaesthesia + adjuvant analgesics (acting peripherally or centrally)
Local anaesthesia + sedation
Local anaesthesia + sedation + adjuvant analgesics (acting peripherally or centrally)
Local anaesthesia + light general anaesthesia
Local anaesthesia + light general anaesthesia + adjuvant analgesics
Balanced analgesia – "multimodal approach" (local anaesthetic block + peripherally acting analgesics + centrally acting analgesics)

---

# Local and regional anaesthesia

Local anaesthesia should be seen as a fundamental working tool, implemented whenever possible in the ambulatory setting. There are a number of different techniques/applications that may be considered for use, independently or in combination (Box 6.2).

Although several types of drugs have been added to local anaesthetics to improve analgesia in inpatients,[13-18] the role of these adjuvants in ambulatory anaesthesia is probably quite limited. One of the main objectives of ambulatory anaesthesia is to allow fast recovery of cognitive and motor function. This may be achieved by adding a small dose of an opioid to the local anaesthetic which will not cause prolonged motor blockade, for example in intraarticular anaesthesia (knee joint, shoulder joint), epidural and spinal anaesthesia (lower extremity surgery). The addition of adrenaline (5 µg/ml) to a local anaesthetic solution serves two purposes: it prolongs the block and it produces vasoconstriction in the surgical field.

## Topical anaesthesia

Most local anaesthetics produce rapid anaesthesia when applied to mucous membranes. It is thus possible to anaesthetise the mouth, pharynx, larynx, trachea, and bronchi. It is also most effective for anaesthesia of the conjunctiva, the nasal cavity, and the urethra.

Topical anaesthesia therefore has a number of indications in ambulatory surgery. Cataract surgery and other surgical procedures on the surface of the ocular bulb are mostly performed under topical anaesthesia. Ear, nose, and throat surgeons usually perform endoscopic and surface procedures

---

**Box 6.2   Local and regional anaesthetic techniques used in ambulatory surgery**

Topical anaesthesia
Infiltration anaesthesia – field blocks
Peripheral nerve blocks
Major peripheral nerve blocks – plexus blocks
Intravenous regional anaesthesia
Central blocks – spinal/epidural

---

under topical anaesthesia. In urological ambulatory surgery, topical anaesthesia can be used for cystoscopy and may also have a place after circumcision for postoperative pain relief.[19] The use of local anaesthesia by EMLA cream or 4% amethocaine ointment in order to facilitate venous access in children should not be neglected.

Topical lignocaine spray applied to the surgical wound has been shown to exert a clear analgesic effect after hysterectomy in a prospective randomised double-blind study.[20]

Instillation of local anaesthesia in the peritoneal cavity during laparoscopic surgery has also been shown to reduce postoperative pain and the need for postoperative analgesics.[21,22]

## Local infiltration or field block

Local infiltration of the surgical area has a central place in all minor superficial surgical procedures. Local anaesthetic infiltration, or field block, has a long history in a variety of more extensive body surface surgery such as inguinal hernia repair and removal of small lumps.

Local anaesthetic infiltration may be used independently or in various combinations (Box 6.1). If the procedure cannot be performed under local anaesthesia only, its supplemental use has a beneficial effect in most instances. The use of locally applied local anaesthesia before the initial incision almost always leads to a decreased need for supplementary intra-operative as well as postoperative opioid analgesics. It may also decrease the need for peroperative anaesthetics. Local anaesthetic infiltration at the end of the procedure has been found useful for postoperative pain relief after surgery performed under either general or regional anaesthesia. From an organisational point of view, local anaesthesia should be used whenever feasible in all ambulatory settings to avoid postoperative pain, because the use of opioids postoperatively will possibly delay discharge.[23,24]

The beneficial effects of local compared to general anaesthesia have been shown for hernia repair and may also be an advantageous alternative for diagnostic arthroscopic procedures.[9,25-29] Local infiltration into the wound for postoperative pain relief has been beneficially applied for all kinds of incisions and procedures, such as in the port sites in arthroscopy and laparoscopy.[30,31] The usefulness of local anaesthetic infiltration of the wound after open inguinal hernia repair, hysterectomy, open cholecystectomy, appendectomy, and various other major surgical procedures has been studied.[32,33]

At present, data showing the statistical significance of the independent beneficial effects of local infiltration are not overwhelming. There are studies showing a decrease in the intensity of postoperative pain, decreased need for analgesics, and shorter time to discharge. Other studies, however, have not been able to confirm these effects.[34] The overall picture seems to be in favour of the use of local anaesthetic infiltration in ambulatory surgery to decrease postoperative pain intensity and need for analgesics, thereby facilitating recovery.[35]

The use of what is nowadays called "balanced analgesia" or "multimodal analgesic technique" (Box 6.1) has a sound theoretical and scientific basis. The combination of local anaesthesia, peripheral acting analgesics such as NSAIDs and central analgesics/anaesthesia has been beneficial not only in the early postoperative period but it also increases the speed of return to ordinary function.[36,37]

Bearing in mind that local anaesthetics are relatively inexpensive and associated with very minor side effects when employed appropriately, surgical wound infiltration with local anaesthetics should be used whenever feasible. Reducing the drugs that may cause sedation, dizziness, and emesis while still providing good postoperative analgesia are key factors in ambulatory anaesthesia. A pain-free patient with intact cognitive function can be safely discharged.

The choice of local anaesthetic should be based on the clinical requirements and pharmacological profile. If time of onset of surgical analgesia is a critical issue, prilocaine or lignocaine would be preferable. When postoperative analgesia is of major importance, the use of bupivacaine or ropivacaine should be advocated, perhaps at the expense of a slightly delayed onset. The addition of adrenaline increases the duration of anaesthesia and analgesia to some extent. However, this should be the surgeon's decision, based on factors such as the anticipated duration of surgery and the vasoconstrictive requirements.

Infiltrating the incisional area with an adequate volume of 10–15 ml of prilocaine or 5 or 10 mg/ml of lignocaine before the start of surgery and an appropriate volume of long-acting local anaesthetic, bupivacaine or ropivacaine 10–20 ml of 2.5 mg/ml, at wound closure is advisable.

A field block in combination with intraarticular administration of prilocaine is common practice before arthroscopic procedures. This technique has replaced the interscalene block for shoulder arthroscopy in many ambulatory centres. At the end of surgery intraarticular instillation of 10–15 ml of bupivacaine 2.5 mg/ml in combination with fentanyl 50 µg or morphine 1–2 mg is often quite effective for postoperative pain relief.

## Peripheral nerve blocks

Peripheral nerve blocks are useful for many procedures. Manual dexterity and experience have an important influence on the success of several of these blocks. This is true particularly when blocks are performed without the aid of a nerve stimulator ("nerve finder"). With the appropriate use of a nerve stimulator, however, even a less experienced anaesthesiologist can identify and block larger nerves.[38] Blocks of the finger and the toe, the ankle, the penis, and the axillary brachial plexus can be achieved with a high success rate without a nerve stimulator.

Ankle block, for instance, is a simple and safe method for foot surgery.[39] It is most effective in decreasing the need for peroperative anaesthetics and analgesics even in patients under general anaesthesia while providing postoperative pain relief for several hours. The tibial nerve and sural nerve are blocked behind both malleoli, while the saphenous nerve and both peroneal (deep and superficial) nerves are blocked at the anterior aspect of the ankle (Fig. 3.7, p. 46). Local anaesthetic without the addition of adrenaline is used for short procedures, for instance lignocaine 10 mg/ml, and for longer ones bupivacaine 5 mg/ml, 3–6 ml at each site (total 15–20 ml).

The penile block is most useful for circumcision.[40] Bupivacaine 5 mg/ml (1–10 ml, according to age and size) produces both good intraoperative conditions and postoperative pain relief for several hours.

Paracervical block is an alternative anaesthetic technique for hysteroscopic procedures.[41] Mepivacaine 5–10 mg/ml 20 ml is usually sufficient for these procedures.

The brachial plexus block is effective for hand surgery; in adults 30–50 ml mepivacaine 10 mg/ml around the brachial artery is usually adequate. In particular, for the supraclavicular plexus approach, the success rate will be increased and performance time reduced when a nerve stimulator is used. The place of supraclavicular blocks of the brachial plexus in the ambulatory setting may be questioned because of the concomitant phrenic nerve block (diaphragmatic paralysis) and the risk of needle-induced pneumothorax.

There are a number of other peripheral blocks with potential usefulness in ambulatory anaesthesia. The use of a nerve block in combination with sedation or light general anaesthesia should always be considered as an alternative technique to general anaesthesia. The fact that it takes some time to acquire skills may be an important limiting factor in a busy practice. A failed block is distressing, firstly to the patient but also to the organisation because of the potential delays as it can take some time to arrange supplementary analgesia or, when necessary, convert to general anaesthesia. Working up routines for performing the various blocks and how to act in the event of a partial or complete failure is necessary. It may be worthwhile supplementing an incomplete block with small analgesic intravenous doses of ketamine, approximately 0.1 mg/kg IV, which gives rapid analgesia with minimal side effects.

As the peripheral blocks will interfere not only with the pain perception but also to some extent with sensory, proprioception, and motor function, many institutions recommend that at least motor function should have resolved before the patient is discharged. Alternatively, patients should be clearly informed of the risks of injury associated with missing sensory or motor nerve functions, for example when arm movements cannot be actively controlled for 5–10 hours after an axillary brachial plexus block.

Recently, catheter techniques for home use have been described both for local infiltration blocks and peripheral blocks, allowing the patient to self-administer low concentrations of local anaesthetic for pain relief.[42] With this technique good postoperative analgesia has been reported without the use of any centrally acting analgesics. Whether this technique will gain popularity in ambulatory anaesthesia remains to be seen. As the level of monitoring and supervision is inferior to that practised in hospital, the detection and treatment of systemic local anaesthetic toxicity in the home environment may be an important problem.

## Intravenous regional anaesthesia – IVRA (Bier's block)

This is an old and simple but still most effective technique for producing anaesthesia of both upper and lower limbs (see Chapter 4). It is based on the fact that when a tourniquet occludes the circulation to a limb and local anaesthetic is injected into a vein distal to the occlusion, the drug will reach the capillaries and diffuse into the tissue, including nerves, by retrograde flow. It will create a block of nerve function distal to the occlusion.

For the arm, 40 ml of a local anaesthetic solution is usually sufficient in adult patients and for the leg, if the cuff is applied around the calf, 40 ml is adequate. The technique is also applicable for analgesia in the foot with a tourniquet placed around the ankle. Preservative-free prilocaine 5 mg/ml is often used, being the least toxic of the available local anaesthetic amides.

Intravenous regional anaesthesia is a most useful alternative anaesthetic techninque for procedures lasting 30–60 minutes. Discomfort from the cuff may be avoided to some extent by the use of a "double cuff" tourniquet. By inflating the proximal cuff initially and switching the pressure to the distal cuff after approximately 20 minutes, this discomfort may be eliminated.

The cuff should not be deflated too early following injection of the local anaesthetic, even if surgery is completed. An early deflation may create high systemic concentrations of local anaesthesia and possibly toxic symptoms. Twenty to 30 minutes is usually sufficient to allow tissue binding of the local anaesthetic and reduce the risk of toxic side effects upon deflation of the tourniquet cuff.

## Central blocks – spinal and epidural anaesthesia

Central blocks are used in most ambulatory centres. The exact role of central block spinal and epidural anaesthesia in ambulatory anaesthesia is still under debate. It is important to consider the goals for ambulatory surgery, i.e. to achieve good intraoperative conditions for the patient and the surgeon but also working towards a fast and complete recovery of all bodily functions.

### Spinal anaesthesia

Spinal anaesthesia is an established anaesthetic technique for procedures on the lower abdomen, perineum, urinary tract, and lower limbs. It is a technique that is easy to adopt and requires limited resources to perform. When applied appropriately, it is associated with a low risk of major sequelae. However, its use in ambulatory anaesthesia is still controversial and its risks should be carefully weighed against its benefits and compared with those of alternative techniques. The risk of spinal haematoma and neural damage is low but these issues have been continuously debated.[43,44]

There are also minor sequelae to consider. The occurrence of postdural puncture headache (PDPH) is one concern. The incidence of PDPH is associated with the size of the needle and the shape of the needle tip.[46] For ambulatory practice, thin (25–27 G) pencil-point needles are most appropriate and PDPH is no longer seen as a major limiting factor.[47] There are also reports of back pain after spinal anaesthesia, which may be related to the local anaesthetic solution. The delayed resumption of bladder function may be a limiting factor in day surgery.

For the inpatient the use of spinal anaesthesia has been shown to have a clear positive benefit versus risk ratio for surgical procedures "below the umbilicus".[45] Whether these results are also applicable in the ambulatory setting and patient population is debatable. There is a lack of studies focusing on hard outcome data, such as major morbidity and mortality, when different anaesthetic techniques are compared for ambulatory procedures. At present, it seems difficult to make any statement regarding the impact of spinal anaesthesia on outcome, bearing in mind the very low overall major morbidity/mortality associated with ambulatory anaesthesia. The choice of spinal anaesthesia seems obvious in patients where general anaesthesia is associated with an increased risk, such as in those who are obese or who have pulmonary disease.

The choice of local anaesthetic is limited by the fact that only a few drugs have been officially registered for intrathecal use. However, almost all available preservative-free local anaesthetic solutions have been used for spinal anaesthesia, For many years lignocaine, mainly hyperbaric lignocaine 50 mg/ml, has been regarded as the drug of choice because of its advantageous pharmacological profile, with a fast onset and offset. Surgical anaesthesia is achieved within minutes and wears off within 1–2 hours. With bupivacaine, the time to surgical anaesthesia is longer, 10–15 min, and the block wears off slowly. Full motor function returns after 3–4 hours and there could be residual bladder dysfunction for a further few hours.[48]

The use of hyperbaric lignocaine 50 mg/ml has been found to be associated with back and radiating leg ache after resolution of the block. Because of the transient nature of these distressing symptoms, they were initially called transient radicular irritation (TRI).[49] One possible cause has been claimed to be direct irritation of the nerve root by the high concentration of lignocaine. However, lignocaine, independent of the concentration and baricity of the solution, seems to be associated with a higher incidence of this syndrome compared to bupivacaine.[50-52] A few cases of even more serious neural damage, i.e. cauda equina, by "single-shot" spinal anaesthesia with concentrated lignocaine have been reported.[53]

Other causes of these symptoms, such as musculoskeletal pain and pain from subdural bleeding, have also been considered. Due to uncertainty regarding the exact mechanism of the radiating aching symptoms, they are now called transient neurological symptoms (TNSs) (see Chapter 8). As a result of the awareness of these problems, several centres now advocate a restriction of the use of hyperbaric lignocaine, as well as of other concentrated local anaesthetic solutions for spinal anaesthesia.

Many attempts have been made to achieve a "fast-resolving" alternative to lignocaine. For instance, small doses and various concentrations of bupivacaine (5-10 mg in adults) have been tried, with some success.[54] The combination of local anaesthetic with a small dose of an opioid intrathecally is an alternative in spinal anaesthesia for minor laparoscopic procedures.[55-57] The use of intrathecal opioids in ambulatory anaesthesia is controversial but the opioid dose is usually very small (10–20 µg fentanyl) and cannot be expected to have any adverse effect on respiration. For inguinal hernia repair, varicose veins and knee arthroscopic procedures, lidocaine 50–60 mg in combination with fentanyl 10 µg usually provides satisfactory anaesthesia. The motor and bladder functions usually resolve within 60–90 min. This technique may be a good alternative to general anaesthesia in appropriate patients.

Viewing the endpoints such as return of body functions, general anaesthesia with the modern agents in combination with an appropriate analgesic strategy may be more advantageous than spinal anaesthesia in certain procedures.[58] On the other hand, there are many surgical procedures where peripheral regional anaesthesia should be considered, as an equal alternative to both general and spinal anaesthesia, and evaluated. For instance, femoral block is an effective alternative to spinal anaesthesia for stripping of the saphenous vein.[59]

Spinal anaesthesia has a definite place in ambulatory anaesthesia but its use should be reevaluated. Factors such as the potential benefits regarding morbidity, no cognitive interference, and extensive analgesia and anaesthesia should be weighed against the risks for minor morbidity, both from the technique itself and those associated with the local anaesthetic solution and the time to resolution of the block.

### Epidural anaesthesia

Epidural anaesthesia with an indwelling catheter is a unique tool for many inpatient surgical procedures. The block may be established prior to surgery in order to decrease the spinal inflow of nociceptive afferent signals and possibly decrease a secondary hyperalgesic response. An extensive sensory block may also reduce the endocrine response associated with the surgical trauma. And last but not least, it may provide excellent postoperative pain relief during the entire postoperative course.[60–63]

Whether these features have implications for ambulatory surgery may be debated. The ongoing increase in medium-large surgical procedures carried out on an outpatient basis may necessitate its use. But as long as the organisational description of ambulatory surgery ends with the statement "It should be limited to less extensive surgery, such as minor laparoscopic procedures", the place of epidural perioperative analgesia can be questioned. Bearing in mind both the extent of ambulatory surgery and the time to discharge, which is of great importance, the use of the epidural catheter technique seems relatively marginal at the present time. However, the use of a "single-shot" epidural block with a rapidly acting local anaesthetic may be seen as an option especially in patients with a high risk of developing PDPH.

In cases of surgery of the lower part of the body in which the duration of surgery is unpredictable, the combined spinal epidural (CSE) technique may also be a choice. Using specially designed CSE sets, both the spinal block and the insertion of the epidural catheter (as a back-up) can be accomplished using the "needle-through-needle" technique in only one vertebral interspace (see Chapter 3).

## Local anaesthesia in ambulatory anaesthesia today and in the future

Ambulatory anaesthesia has grown tremendously in numbers of cases and in quality during the last decade and this expansion is set to continue.[3] Ambulatory anaesthesia is associated with very low mortality and morbidity.[5] This is probably due to the facts that only minor to medium-large surgery has been performed and that the patient population almost exclusively belong to the ASA I – II class.[3,5] One can imagine that in the near future, the surgical procedures will be slightly more extensive in an older patient population carrying a far more complex medical history.[64] This will call for vigilant anaesthetic attention. The techniques and drugs used should be analysed and evaluated appropriately and repeatedly to meet the changing and challenging needs of ambulatory anaesthesia.

The concept of balanced analgesia (the multimodal approach) has become a gold standard in ambulatory anaesthesia. Combining local-regional anaesthesia with peripherally acting systemic analgesics if necessary, with additional small doses of opioids and/or sedation with fast-acting hypnotics such as propofol, plays a central role in ambulatory anaesthesia today.[65] One can also predict that in the future local-regional anaesthesia, NSAIDs, and paracetamol with a peripheral action will form the platform for analgesia in the perioperative period of ambulatory surgery.[30,66,67] An improvement in selectivity and duration of action of the local anaesthetics would further increase the clinical advantage of local-regional anaesthesia in ambulatory surgery.[68]

It remains to be evaluated whether a peripheral catheter technique for repeated administration of local anaesthetics by the patient ("patient-controlled regional analgesia") after discharge will have a place in clinical ambulatory surgery.

1 Woolf C. Recent advances in the pathophysiology of acute pain. *Br J Anaesth* 1989;**63**:139–46.
2 Woolf CJ. Generation of acute pain: central mechanisms. *Br Med Bull* 1991;**47**:523–33.
3 Osborne GA, Rudkine GE. Outcome after day-care surgery in a major teaching hospital. *Anaesth Intens Care* 1993;**21**:822–7.
4 Marshall S, Chung F. Discharge criteria and complications after ambulatory surgery. *Anesth Analg* 1999;**88**:508–17.
5 Warner MA, Shields SE, Chute CG. Major morbitity and mortality within 1 month of ambulatory surgery and anesthesia. *JAMA* 1993;**270**:1437–41.
6 Chung F. Recovery pattern and home-readiness after ambulatory surgery. *Anaesth Analg* 1995;**80**:896–902.
7 Gold B, Kitz D, Lecky J, Neuhaus J. Unanticipated admission to the hospital following ambulatory surgery. *JAMA* 1989;**262**:3008–10.
8 Tzabar Y, Asbury AJ, Millar K. Cognitive failure after general anaesthesia for day case surgery. *Br J Anaesth* 1996;**76**:194–7.
9 Teasdale C, McCrum AM, Williams NB, Horton RE. A randomised controlled trial to compare local with general anaesthesia for short-stay inguinal hernia repair. *Ann R Coll Surg Engl* 1982;**64**:238–42.
10 Tzabar Y, Asbury AJ, Millar K. Cognitive failure after general anaesthesia for day case surgery. *Br J Anaesth* 1996;**76**:194–7.

11 Phillips B. Supplemental medication for ambulatory procedures under regional anesthesia. *Anesth Analg* 1985;**64**:1117–25.

12 White PF, Song D. New criteria for fast-tracking after outpatient anesthesia: a comparison with the modified Aldrete's scoring system. *Anesth Analg* 1999;**88**:1069–72.

13 O'Hanlon JJ, McClean G, Muldoon T. Preoperative application of piroxicam gel compared to a local anaesthesia field block for postoperative analgesia. *Acta Anaesthesiol Scand* 1996;**40**:715–18.

14 Cook TM, Tuckey JP, Nolan JP. Analgesia after day-case arthroscopy: double-blind study of intra-articular tenoxicam, intra-articular bupivacaine and placebo. *Br J Anaesth* 1997;**78**:163–8.

15 Varrassi G, Marinangeli F, Ciccozzi A, Iovinelli G, Facchetti G, Ciccone A. Intra-articular buprenorphine after knee arthroscopy. A randomised, prospective, double-blind study. *Acta Anaesthesiol Scand* 1999;**43**:51–5.

16 Chia Y-Y, Liu Y-C, Chang H-C, Wong CS. Efficacy of ketamine in multimodal epidural analgesia. *Anesth Analg* 1998;**86**:1245–9.

17 De Kock M, Wiederkher P, Laghmiche A, Scholtes J-L. Epidural clonidine used as the sole analgesic agent during and after abdominal surgery. *Anesthesiology* 1997;**86**:185–92.

18 Cheng Yang L, Chen L-M, Wang C-J, Buerkle H. Postoperative analgesia by intra-articular neostigmine in patients undergoing knee arthroscopy. *Anesthesiology* 1998;**88**:334–9.

19 Nazarali S, Muttitt S. Comparison of ring block, dorsal penile nerve block, and topical anesthesia for neonatal circumcision: a randomized controlled trial. *JAMA* 1997;**278**:2157–62.

20 Sinclair R, Westlander G, Cassuto J, Hedner T. Postoperative pain relief by topical lidocaine in the surgical wound of hysterectomized patients. *Acta Anaesthesiol Scand* 1996;**40**:589–94.

21 Pasqualucci A, de Angelis V, Contardo R et al. Preemptive analgesia: intraperitoneal local anesthetic in laparoscopic cholecystectomy. *Anesthesiology* 1996;**85**:11–20.

22 Callesen T, Hjort D, Schouenborg L, Nielsen D, Reventlid H, Kehlet H. Combined field block and i.p. instillation of ropivacaine for pain management after laparoscopic sterilization. *Br J Anaesth* 1999;**82**:586–90.

23 Jakobsson J, Davidson S, Andreen M, Westgren M. Opioid supplementation to propofol anaesthesia for outpatient abortion: a comparison between alfentanil, fentanyl and placebo. *Acta Anaesthesiol Scand* 1991;**35**:767–70.

24 Jakobsson J, Oddby E, Rane K. Patient evaluation of four different combinations of intravenous anaesthetics for short outpatient procedures. *Anaesthesia* 1993;**48**:1005–7.

25 Subramaniam P, Leslie J, Gourlay C, Clezy JK. Inguinal hernia repair: a comparison between local and general anaesthesia. *Aust NZ J Surg* 1998;**68**:799–800.

26 Schumpelick V, Peiper C, Tons C, Kupczyk-Joeris D, Busch F. Inguinal hernia repair with local anesthesia – a comparative analysis. *Langenbecks Arch Chir* 1993;**378**:329–34.

27 Peiper C, Tons C, Schippers E, Busch F, Schumpelick V. Local versus general anesthesia for Shouldice repair of the inguinal hernia. *World J Surg* 1994;**18**:912–16.

28 Williams CR, Thomas NP. A prospective trial of local versus general anaesthesia for arthroscopic surgery of the knee. *Ann R Coll Surg Engl* 1997;**79**:345–8.

29  Lintner S, Shawen S, Lohnes J, Levy A, Garrett W. Local anesthesia in outpatient knee arthroscopy: a comparison of efficacy and cost. *Arthroscopy* 1996;**12**:482–8.

30  Morrow BC, Milligan KR, Murthy BVS. Analgesia following day-case arthroscopy – the effect of piroxicam with or without bupivacaine infiltration. *Anaesthesia* 1995;**50**:461–3.

31  Callesen T, Hjort D, Schouenborg L, Nielsen D, Reventlid H, Kehlet H. Combined field block and i.p. instillation of ropivacaine for pain management after laparoscopic sterilization. *Br J Anaesth* 1999;**82**:586–90.

32  Dierking GW, Dahl JB, Kanstrup J, Dahl A, Kehlet H. Effect of pre- vs postoperative inguinal field block on postoperative pain after herniorrhaphy. *Br J Anaesth* 1992;**68**:334–48.

33  Dierking GW, Ostergaard E, Ostergard HT, Dahl JB. The effects of wound infiltration with bupivacaine versus saline on postoperative pain and opioid requirements after herniorrhaphy. *Acta Anaesthesiol Scand* 1994;**38**:289–92.

34  Dahl J, Moiniche S, Kehlet H. Wound infiltration with local anaesthetics for postoperative pain relief. *Acta Anaesthesiol Scand* 1994;**38**:7–14.

35  Moiniche S, Mikkelsen S, Wetterslev, Dahl JB. A quantitative systematic review of incisional local anaesthesia for postoperative pain relief after abdominal operations. *Br J Anaesth* 1998;**81**:377–83.

36  Eriksson H, Tenhunen A, Korttila K. Balanced analgesia improves recovery and outcome after outpatient tubal ligation. *Acta Anaesthesiol Scand* 1996;**40**:151–5.

37  Michaloliakou C, Chung F, Sharma S. Preoperative multimodal analgesia facilitates recovery after ambulatory laparoscopic cholecystectomy. *Anesth Analg* 1996;**82**:44–51.

38  Koscielniak-Nielsen ZJ, Rotboll Nielsen P, Loumann Nielsen S, Gardi T, Hermann C. Comparison of transarterial and multiple nerve stimulation techniques for axillary block using a high dose of mepivacaine with adrenaline. *Acta Anaesthesiol Scand* 1999;**43**:398–404.

39  Tryba M. Ankle block: a safe and simple technique for foot surgery. *Curr Opin Anaesthesiol* 1997;**10**:361–5.

40  Seour F, Cohen A, Mandelberg A, Mori J, Ezra S. Dorsal penile nerve block in children undergoing circumcision in a day-care surgery. *Can J Anaesth* 1996;**43**:954–8.

41  Anathanarayan C, Paek W, Rolbin S, Dhanidina K. Hysteroscopy and anaesthesia. *Can J Anaesth* 1996;**43**:56–64.

42  Rawal N, Axelsson K, Hylander J et al. Postoperative patient-controlled local anesthetic administration at home. *Anesth Analg* 1998;**86**:86–9.

43  Breivik H. Neurological complications in association with spinal and epidural analgesia – again. *Acta Anaesthesiol Scand* 1998;**42**:609–13.

44  Dahlgren N, Törnebrandt K. Neurological complications after anaesthesia. A follow-up of 18 000 spinal and epidural anaesthetics performed over three years. *Acta Anaesthesiol Scand* 1995;**39**:872–80.

45  Scott NB, Kehlet H. Regional anaesthesia and surgical morbidity. *Br J Surg* 1988;**75**:299–304.

46  Halpern S, Preston R. Postdural puncture headache and spinal needle design. Metaanalyses. *Anesthesiology* 1994;**81**:1376–83.

47  Eriksson AL, Hallen B, Persson E, Sköldefors E. Whitacre or Quincke needles – does it really matter? *Acta Anaesthesiol Scand* 1998;**42**:17–20.

48  Kamphuis ET, Ionescu TI, Kuipers PW, de Gier J, van Venrooij Ge, Boon TA.

Recovery of storage and emptying function of the urinary bladder after spinal anesthesia with lidocaine and with bupivacaine in man. *Anesthesiology* 1998;**88**:310–16.

49 Schneider M, Ettlin T, Kaufmann M *et al.* Transient neurologic toxicity after hyperbaric subarachnoid anesthesia with 5% lidocaine. *Anesth Analg* 1993;**76**:1154–7.

50 Hampl KF, Heinzmann-Wiedmer S, Luginbuehl I *et al.* Transient neurological symptoms after spinal anesthesia. A lower incidence with prilocaine and bupivacaine than with lidocaine. *Anesthesiology* 1998;**88**:629–33

51 Freedman JM, Li D-K, Drasner K, Jaskela M, Larsen B, Wi S. Transient neurological symptoms after spinal anesthesia. An epidemiological study of 1863 patients. *Anesthesiology* 1998;**89**:633–41.

52 Liguori G, Zayas V, Chisholm M. Transient neurological symptoms after spinal anesthesia with mepivacaine and lidocaine. *Anesthesiology* 1998;**88**:619–23.

53 Loo C, Irestedt L. Cauda equina syndrome after spinal anaesthesia with hyperbaric 5% lidocain: a review of six cases of cauda equina syndrome reported to the Swedish Pharmaceuticaal Insurance 1993–1997. *Acta Anaesthesiol Scand* 1999;**43**:371–9.

54 Ben-David B, Levin H, Solomon E *et al.* Spinal bupivacaine in ambulatory surgery: the effect of saline dilution. *Anesth Analg* 1996;**83**:716–20.

55 Ben-David B, Solomon E, Levin H, Admoni H, Goldik Z. Intrathecal fentanyl with small-dose diluted bupivacaine: better anesthesia without prolonging recovery. *Anesth Analg* 1997;**85**:560–5.

56 Vaghadia H, McLeod D, Mitchell E, Merrick P, Chilvers C. Small-dose hypobaric lidocaine-fentanyl spinal anesthesia for short duration outpatient laparoscopy. I. A randomized comparison with conventional hyperbaric lidocaine. *Anesth Analg* 1997;**84**:59–64.

57 Chilvers CR, Vaghadia H, Mitchell GW, Merrick PM. Small-dose hypobaric lidocaine-fentanyl spinal anaesthesia for short duration outpatient laparoscopy. II. Optimal fentanyl dose. *Anesth Analg* 1997;**84**:65–70.

58 Dahl V, Gieroff C, Omland E, Raeder JC. Spinal, epidural or propofol anaesthesia for out-patient knee arthrosopy. *Acta Anaesthesiol Scand* 1997;**41**:1341–5.

59 Vloka JD, Hadzic A, Mulcare R, Lesser JB, Kitain E, Thys DM. Femoral and genitofemoral nerve blocks versus spinal anesthesia for outpatients undergoing long saphenous vein stripping. *Anesth Analg* 1997;**84**:749–52.

60 McQueen DA, Kelly HK, Wright TF. A comparison of epidural and nonepidural anesthesia and analgesia in total hip or knee arthroplasty patients. *Orthopedics* 1992;**15**:169–73.

61 Moiniche S, Hjortso NC, Hansen BL *et al.* The effect of balanced analgesia on early convalescence after major orthopaedic surgery. *Acta Anaesthesiol Scand* 1994;**38**:328–35.

62 Watson A, Allen PR. Influence of thoracic epidural analgesia on outcome after resection for esophageal cancer. *Surgery* 1994;**115**:429–32.

63 Parker SD, Breslow MJ, Frank SM *et al.* Ischemia Randomized Anesthesia Trial Study Group. Catecholamine and cortisol responses to lower extremity revascularization: correlation with outcome variables. *Crit Care Med* 1995;**23**:1954–61.

64 Vaghadia H. Outpatient anesthesia. Some aging perspectives: advice from a caterpillar. *Can J Anaesth* 1999;**46**:305–8.

65 Pavlin DJ, Rapp SE, Polissar NL *et al.* Factors affecting discharge time in adult outpatients. *Anaesth Analg* 1998;**87**:816–26.

66  Ben-David B, Baune-Goldstein U, Goldik Z, Gaitini L. Is preoperative ketorolac a useful adjunct to regional anesthesia for inguinal herniorrhaphy? *Acta Anaesthesiol Scand* 1996;**40**:358–65.
67  Nehra D, Gemmell L, Pye JK. Pain relief after inguinal hernia repair: a randomized double-blind study. *Br J Surg* 1995;**82**:1245–7.
68  Renck H. Wound infiltration with local anaesthetics. *Acta Anaesthesiol Scand* 1994;**38**:2–6.

# 7: Epidural and spinal anaesthesia and analgesia in obstetrics

MARCEL VERCAUTEREN

During the last decade several developments have increased the safety of perinatal analgesia and anaesthesia. Technical innovations and new drugs have invited many investigators to search for improvements, the benefits of which have not always been easy to demonstrate, however. As labour pain has received the greatest attention, this overview will mainly focus on labour analgesia rather than caesarean section anaesthesia and analgesia. All recent developments in neuraxial analgesia can be discussed in relationship to their increased safety and beneficial effect upon the progress of labour.

## Obstetrical outcome

The effect of epidural analgesia upon instrumental delivery (ID) and/or caesarean section (CS) rate has been a controversial issue for decades, as epidural analgesic block may be a marker of an abnormal labour rather than the cause of it. Dystocia may cause more pain whereas pain may induce dysfunctional labour. Epidural analgesia is more frequently requested by nulliparous parturients, during long-lasting, exhaustive labour or trial of labour. Only by performing randomised trials, avoiding a population bias, may final evidence be obtained.

Despite ethical concerns, the first to perform such a randomised study during both labour stages were Thorp et al,[1] who studied 200 patients receiving either bupivacaine 0.25% followed by an infusion with 0.125% bupivacaine or systemic pethidine (meperidine)/promethazine. They found longer labour, more oxytocin requirements, and a higher CS rate (25% vs 2%), mostly for dystocia, in patients receiving epidural analgesia. This study raised many comments criticising the non-blinding of the obstetricians in their decision making, the poorly detailed analgesic protocol, the premature termination of the study, their different data in comparison with those of other centres and the longer delay in the epidural group between admittance, randomisation, and initiation of pain treatment. Their suggestion to initiate epidural analgesia only after cervical dilatation had reached 5 cm was contested by two studies by Chestnut et al in both spontaneous and induced labour.[2,3]

The problem of labour progress and epidural analgsia has been tackled in larger and more recent studies. In the first study in 1330 women, epidural bupivacaine/fentanyl was compared with intravenous pethidine.[4] In both groups one out of three parturients did not receive the allocated treatment as 35% of the patients in the first group did not receive epidural analgesia whereas in the pethidine group 103 women (i.e. 15%) requested epidural analgesia because of insufficient pain relief. Another 19% of the latter group was not treated as intended. Outcome according to 'compliance' revealed a significant decrease from a 9% incidence of CS in the epidural group to 4% in the pethidine group. However, the exclusion of one out of three of their patients might have affected this difference as parturients having an easy labour did not receive epidural analgesia whereas those in the pethidine group having a difficult labour received epidural analgesia afterwards.

This forced the authors to perform a second study in 715 women but taking into account the original randomisation.[5] Again, around 30% did not complete the study as allocated. Intention-to-treat analysis did not demonstrate any difference with respect to CS or forceps delivery rate. This second study taught that intravenous patient-controlled analgesia (PCA) with pethidine is an excellent alternative, offering much satisfaction in spite of the fact that mothers were more sedated and more neonates required naloxone.

Recently, it was shown that epidural analgesia may induce maternal fever, being responsible for a higher incidence of CS rate and neonatal septic work-ups.[6-8] Further randomised studies have been initiated meanwhile to provide final evidence with respect to the effect of analgesia, parity, fever, induction, and duration of labour upon instrumental delivery/C-section. Preliminary results suggest that factors other than epidural analgesia per se are involved. Several methods have been initiated to minimise this effect upon outcome, such as the addition of opioids, epidural PCA (PCEA), newer local anaesthetics, combined spinal and epidural block (CSE) and continuous spinal anaesthesia (CSA) techniques, ambulation, and elective CS upon request.

## Addition of analgesic substances to epidural bupivacaine

When an opioid is added to a potent bolus dose of bupivacaine, the duration of pain relief may be doubled. Alternatively the concentration of the local anaesthetic (LA) may be decreased. Both approaches offer more safety to both mother and neonate as less LA will be required per total labour time. This will cause less relaxation of the pelvic floor, enabling proper rotation and descent of the foetal head. During the second stage this concentration may offer a compromise between satisfactory analgesia, preservation of the bearing down reflex, and maternal motor power for expulsion. Recently, two large randomised studies were able to show fewer ID in patients receiving bupivacaine 0.125% with sufentanil 1 µg/ml as opposed to groups receiving the local anaesthetic alone.[9,10]

Although any opioid could be used, fentanyl and sufentanil are the most popular opioids combined with bupivacaine for labour analgesia. Fentanyl concentrations range from 1 to 2.5 µg/ml, 2 µg/ml being the average, following loading doses of 25–100 µg. In epidural use, sufentanil is known to be 3–5 times more potent than fentanyl. Therefore sufentanil, when added at 1 µg/ml, may signify a relative overdose whereas 0.5–0.75 µg/ml seems more appropriate.[11] Loftus et al showed that the foetal/maternal ratio was higher with sufentanil but that due to its lower maternal plasma concentrations, placental transfer was minimal.[12] As a consequence, detectable levels of sufentanil were measured in fewer umbilical artery blood samples than after administration of fentanyl and neuroadaptive scores were better in the sufentanil-bupivacaine group than in the fentanyl-bupivacaine and bupivacaine-alone groups after 24 hours.

Clonidine may also be added to local anaesthetics. Claes et al[13] demonstrated that the addition of clonidine to a mixture of bupivacaine, adrenaline, and sufentanil resulted in 75% reduction of required epidural bupivacaine as compared to bupivacaine alone and improved quality of analgesia, while offering a higher degree of satisfaction than the other mixtures. However, the higher incidence of hypotension and sedation after the epidural clonidine-containing mixture may compromise the future popularity of clonidine for labour analgesia.

## Patient-controlled epidural analgesia

Using the same principles and equipment as in the intravenous analgesia technique called patient-controlled analgesia (PCA), the patient can also self-administer analgesic agents through an epidural catheter for the control of pain. PCEA may offer several advantages as compared to bolus injections. Because the time between reappearance of pain and treatment will be reduced, parturients may be more satisfied. With regard to safety, intrathecal catheter migration may be self-limiting as parturients will experience excellent pain relief while complaining of motor block which, logically, does not correlate with the dose of bupivacaine administered. Unintentional intravascular injection, on the other hand, will result in increasing pain earlier than toxic symptoms provided that low concentrations and doses are used. In the PCEA technique, the risk of injecting the wrong substance is also less than with bolus injections.

When comparing the intermittent bolus top-up administration technique with PCEA, several studies have found equal consumption with both techniques without any further difference except improved satisfaction.[14,15] Two other studies found a small but significant dose sparing in favour of PCEA with comparable satisfaction when the top-up provider is permanently present on the obstetrical ward.[16,17] Compared to continuous epidural infusion (CEI), PCEA treatment with or without background infusion may offer a significant dose-sparing effect.[15,16,18] With epidural opioids alone, postoperative pain studies have demonstrated that a basal rate will only increase the consumption of the narcotic and the incidence of side effects without improving the quality of analgesia.[19] However, obstetric pain is quite different because epidural opioids alone will be unable to treat pain sufficiently unless local anaesthetics are added. Ferrante et al found analgesia to be better when providing a basal epidural infusion rate, a 6 ml/h rate requiring fewer interventions by the anaesthetist than a 3 ml/h basal rate.[18] However, it may be expected that the higher the amount of the concurrent infusion, the smaller the difference between the efficacy of PCEA and CEI.

Volumes delivered by PCEA pumps are rather small and should not exceed 5–6 ml per demand dose. Therefore extremely weak concentrations in PCEA are less practical as they would require either excessive volumes, (too) high opioid doses or combination with adjuvant drugs such as clonidine. Ferrante et al found a 35% dose sparing when using bupivacaine 0.125% + fentanyl 2 µg/ml in PCEA as compared to CEI.[18] Decreasing the bupivacaine concentration in PCEA to 0.0625% with identical PCEA settings did not result in further dose reductions, demonstrating that more demands were necessary.[20]

## Ropivacaine/levobupivacaine

As opposed to racemic bupivacaine, ropivacaine and levobupivacaine are almost pure S-enantiomers and may replace bupivacaine because of a safer toxicity profile (see Chapter 1). Most of the recent studies have been performed with ropivacaine. It was believed that ropivacaine would show a greater separation between sensory and motor blocking activity. However, only one out of three studies was able to demonstrate less motor block with ropivacaine while in some the duration of sensory blockade was shorter than with the same concentration of bupivacaine.

A metaanalysis by Writer et al showed that studies comparing bupivacaine and ropivacaine 0.25% for labour analgesia resulted in a similar quality of analgesia but less motor block and ID with the newer substance.[21] Owen *et al*, on the other hand, were unable to find any significant difference when comparing the 0.125% concentration for ropivacaine and bupivacaine.[22] Whereas all these studies were performed with plain solutions, Gautier *et al* showed that the 0.125% concentration combined with sufentanil resulted in findings similar to those revealed by the metaanalysis.[23]

Although it is still believed that the dose-response curve of ropivacaine when compared to bupivacaine is shifted to the right, especially with respect to motor blockade and to a lesser extent for the sensory effect, two recent studies using a similar design have shown, by calculating the $ED_{50}$ doses, that ropivacaine is 40% less potent than bupivacaine.[24,25] As a consequence, the discussion with respect to motor effects and toxicity has to be reconsidered. Cardiac toxicity may still be avoided when using ropivacaine but central nervous toxicity may be more pronounced when equipotent doses of ropivacaine are administered, explaining the possible occurrence of seizures with this drug.

Levobupivacaine is less cardiotoxic compared to bupivacaine but more studies are required to determine the lethal dose, effects on motor block, and central nervous system toxicity.

As in modern labour analgesia low-dose regimens are becoming more popular and cardiac arrest has not been reported during the last 15 years, cost/benefit considerations may call into question whether replacement of bupivacaine during labour is justified after all. Most probably, ropivacaine may be more indicated for caesarean section because of its lower cardiac toxicity when injecting higher doses (i.e. approximately 150 mg) than in labour conditions and would also be beneficial in offering faster recovery of motor function.

## Intrathecal analgesia

Intrathecal administration as part of a combined spinal epidural (CSE) technique may provide effective pain relief.

### Quality of analgesia

Onset of pain relief will be faster than with a pure epidural technique. Analgesia will be bilateral and the quality may be better during the first 20–30 minutes but after this time no major differences have been noticed. The duration of analgesia depends on the stage of labour and the drug or combination injected.[26] Prolongation of lipophilic opioid analgesia has been demonstrated by adding bupivacaine 1–2.5 mg, clonidine 30 µg, adrenaline 25–200 µg or morphine 0.25 mg.[27–29] Table 7.1 shows the duration of the most commonly used drugs and combinations. The longest duration, i.e. >3 hours, has been found with a bupivacaine 2.5 mg-adrenaline 200 μg-sufentanil 10 μg mixture.[28] Since the $ED_{50}$ dose of sufentanil has been found to be 1.8 μg in nulliparous women and 2.6 μg in a mixed population,[30,31] lower doses of opioids, especially in mixtures, may offer excellent pain relief while reducing the risk of side effects.[27, 32, 33]

Table 7.1  Durations of analgesia obtained after intrathecal injection of the most popular substances and combinations during labour (average or ranges)

| Intrathecal opioid and combination | Average duration of analgesia (min) |
| --- | --- |
| Sufentanil 10 μg | 96–124 |
| Fentanyl 25 μg + morphine 0.25 mg | 90 |
| Sufentanil 10 μg + morphine 0.25 mg | 135 |
| Sufentanil 10 μg + epinephrine 200 μg | 132 |
| Fentanyl 25 μg + bupivacaine 2.5 mg | 80–90 |
| Sufentanil 10 μg + bupivacaine 2.5 mg | 120–163 |
| Sufentanil 10 μg + bupivacaine 2.5 mg + adrenaline 200 μg | 188 |
| Sufentanil 5 μg + bupivacaine 1 mg | 110 |
| Sufentanil 5 μg + bupivacaine 1 mg + adrenaline 25 μg | 138–142 |
| Sufentanil 5 μg + clonidine 30 μg | 126–145 |
| Sufentanil 1.2 μg + bupivacaine 2 mg + adrenaline 2 μg | 103 |

Even if not all anaesthetists agree on the superiority of intrathecal analgesia, a CSE technique may be particularly useful in some clinical conditions, as listed in Box 7.1. However, in a 'trial of labour' it may be preferable to use a properly functioning epidural catheter rather than an initial subarachnoid effect but with an untested epidural catheter.

---

**Box 7.1   Possible indications for the use of intrathecal analgesia for the control of labour pain**

- Accidental dural puncture
- Advanced labour (cervical dilatation >5 cm)
- Unbearable pain
- Trial of labour (this indication should be evaluated further)
- Previous back surgery or epidural blood patch (epidural analgesia may not be possible)
- Allergy to local anaesthetics

---

### Safety for mother and foetus

Hypotension may occur following intrathecal injection of opioids. This may be a purely pharmacodynamic effect but it may also be related to the decreased cathecholamine levels during installation of analgesia. A dual effect as with pethidine, i.e. a local anaesthetic and an opiate receptor-mediated one, is probably not present with other opioids.

Lipophilic opioids seem to migrate rostrally, although not to the same extent as less lipid-soluble ones. Intrathecal doses ranging between 10 and 15 μg (more than the recommended epidural dose of 7.5 μg/10 ml bolus) may induce swallowing problems, somnolence, and respiratory depression.[34-37] Nausea and vomiting cannot be avoided and these side effects are both drug and dose dependent.

Dose-dependent pruritus is the most frequent side effect of intrathecal opioid analgesia.[27] With either sufentanil 10 μg or fentanyl 25 μg, the incidence is usually higher than 85%.

Complications related to the CSE technique are accidental dural perforation with the epidural needle, paraesthesiae, and backache but it is not clear whether they are more frequent in obstetric patients. In a large retrospective study, Norris et al did not find any major difference in complication rate between patients treated with CSE, epidural or no neuraxial technique at all.[38]

Meningitis has been reported several times.[39-40] The higher incidence after labour analgesia is probably more related to the less aseptic environment of the labour ward in comparison with operating theatre conditions, than to the CSE technique per se.

Leighton et al found higher dermatomal spread following the first epidural "top-up" dose compared with patients not receiving a dural puncture, which may be explained by drug transfer through the dural hole.[41] This may raise the question whether it is safe to initiate a continuous infusion or PCEA soon after a CSE technique. Collis et al demonstrated that midwife "top-ups" given on request resulted in lower dose requirements than continuous infusion and PCEA whereas a higher degree of safety may be expected when manually administering a bolus dose.[16]

There are several reports of uterine hyperactivity and foetal heart rate changes with CSE analgesia.[42-44] Gambling et al found more caesarean sections for profound bradycardia within the first hour after intrathecal sufentanil administration compared with intravenous pethidine.[45] However, randomised comparative studies could not provide any evidence for a difference between both neuraxial techniques but only noticed that episodes of abnormal foetal heart rates may occur faster with spinally induced pain relief.[46-48] Due to the rapidity of the analgesic effect a disproportional drop of plasma catecholamines may induce uterine hypertonicity, which may be abolished by nitroglycerine.

## Effect upon motor block, instrumental deliveries, and caesarean section

The bupivacaine dose-sparing principle may result in less motor weakness. However, only two out of the nine studies comparing CSE with epidural analgesia were able to find a lower incidence of ID.[46–54] The small sample size of most studies did not allow straightforward conclusions with respect to instrumentation or operative delivery despite significant dose reductions. D'Angelo *et al* found epidural bupivacaine dose reductions exceeding 50 mg during the first stage of labour after 10 μg intrathecal sufentanil, instead of intrathecal saline, but a total epidural dose of >80 mg bupivacaine will still cause muscle relaxation, which may affect the second stage of labour.[51] Others have found only a 9 mg difference between CSE and a low-dose epidural block, which should not have major clinical implications.[52]

The use of ropivacaine by the intrathecal route is very tempting when assuming that equipotent doses may offer less motor impairment than bupivacaine. Ropivacine doses ranging from 2 to 4 mg seem to induce comparable sensory blocks and motor impairment as bupivacaine 2.5 mg, while doses ranging from 0.5 to 2 mg do not induce any clinically observable motor block.[55,56]

### Continuous spinal anaesthesia

Continuous spinal anaesthesia (CSA) will provide excellent bilateral and titratable pain relief but it is not popular for labour analgesia despite the promising initial experience in the early 1990s. Headache, transient neurological complications, cauda equina syndrome, and concerns about the use of microcatheters have diminished or interrupted the practice with this tempting alternative. In addition, the use of continuous intrathecal analgesia with sufentanil 10 μg increments has been found to result in tachyphylaxis or a fading analgesic effect with proceeding uterine cervical dilatation.[57] In a recent preliminary report on CSA in labour, the incidence of epidural blood patch for postural-dependent PDPH was as high as 4%.[58]

# Ambulation during labour

### Advantages

Walking during labour has always been common practice but monitoring, oxytocin augmentation, and neuraxial analgesia have forced patients to return to the horizontal position.

From 1993 on, terms such as "ambulatory", "walking" and "stand-up" labour analgesia were introduced. Meanwhile, many studies have evaluated the safety and possible benefits of ambulation during neuraxial relief of labour pain. Unfortunately, several advantages related to ambulation have been demonstrated only to a limited extent.

*Shorter labour* causes *less pain,* making the parturient more willing to walk and less pain may cause less dysfunctional labour. One report found *fewer caesarean sections* in an ambulating group receiving CSE (8%) compared with an epidural group (42%) not allowed to walk. However, CSE by the low-dose principle, rather than ambulation itself, may explain this difference.[54]

*Better cardiovascular stability* may be obtained while patients walk than with the left lateral or sitting position.[59] Although no correlation could be found between the position and the incidence of hypotension, *improved foetal heart rate recordings* were found while injecting in the standing position in comparison with other postures.

It has been suggested that walking may reduce the incidence of chronic back pain, urinary retention (patients may void on a toilet), and thromboembolic complications but none of these has been clearly demonstrated.

The latest studies in more than 500 parturients not receiving neuraxial pain relief and 229 parturients following CSE analgesia could not show any benefit of maternal ambulation.[60, 61]

Several side effects may be decreased when focusing on low-dose and fine-tuning epidural analgesia and may have nothing to do with ambulation itself. Parturients are probably *more satisfied* with the lack of motor impairment than with the act of walking per se.

### Conditions for allowing ambulation during labour

Several conditions need to be fulfilled before a parturient can be allowed to ambulate (Box 7.2). Patients should be able to raise their straight legs and make a moderate knee-bend. Recently, more attention has been

---

**Box 7.2   Conditions for ambulation during labour under neuraxial analgesia**

- Approval by obstetrician, anaesthetist, and nurse
- Stable vital signs in the erect position for at least 30 min
- No motor block
- Intact proprioception
- No foetal heart rate abnormalities during the first 30 min after analgesic drug injection
- Patients should feel confident to walk
- Restricted area for ambulation
- Assistance during ambulation (2 persons or 1 person + infusion pole)
- Precautions against catheter dislodgement
- Telemetry or returning every 15–30 min for evaluation of cardiotocography

---

focused upon the importance of intact proprioception which should be evaluated by the Romberg test, vibration sense, and joint/muscle proprioception tests. In a maternal ambulation study, Buggy and co-workers found that proprioception was disturbed in the majority of patients receiving a large epidural loading dose (test dose + 15 ml bupivacaine 0.1% + 30 µg fentanyl, followed by an infusion of bupivacaine 0.1% + fentanyl 2 µg/ml) which, however, offered suboptimal analgesia.[62] In a subsequent study the authors showed that an initial dose of 15 ml bupivacaine 0.1% with fentanyl 100 µg provided excellent pain relief and enabled all patients to walk.[63] Parry et al[64] compared epidural analgesia with CSE analgesia (bupivacaine 2.5 mg + fentanyl 25 µg) and found no differences. In both groups of 30 patients each, three were unable to walk while two out of these three experienced proprioceptive deficit.

## Do we need to breach the dura?

Despite the belief that ambulation can be made possible by utilising an intrathecal pain relief method, the first study to report ambulation compared epidural fentanyl (bolus + infusion) with a mixture of bupivacaine 0.04% and fentanyl 1.7 µg/ml by epidural infusion.[65] Since it is difficult to make a clear distinction between the benefit induced by either the ambulation, the low dose CSE or the epidural regimen, the main goal in current labour analgesia is to reduce motor impairment as well as the risk of toxicity. Therefore any low-dose regimen may reduce many of the side effects while offering better chances for natural childbirth. The mother feels when and how to push while being able to preserve expulsive motor capacity. Possible muscle weakness may cause relaxation of the pelvic floor and increase the risk of dystocia and malpresentation.

Several possibilities exist to achieve this goal. CSE/CSA techniques are excellent choices but the use of opioids alone will usually provide pain relief for less than two hours. Addition of bupivacaine, adrenaline or clonidine to the opioid may extend this duration. However, clonidine may increase the risk of hypotension and has not been studied in ambulating parturients while bupivacaine 2.5 mg may not guarantee intact motor function and proprioception in all parturients.[31,64]

Several other studies have demonstrated that ambulation does not necessarily require dural puncturing and subarachnoid drug deposition.[10,53,66] Price et al found that more patients were able to ambulate at 30 min after a low-dose epidural analgesia than a CSE technique but at 60 min no differences were noticed.[53] The lowest effective concentration may be the safest to allow ambulation. If halving the concentration will double the volume required, then no further benefit should be expected from diluting the local anaesthetic too extensively.

A recent comparison between 0.08% ropivacaine versus bupivacaine, both in combination with fentanyl, demonstrated that all patients receiving ropivacaine could ambulate and void while this was impossible in approximately 25% of bupivacaine-treated subjects.[67]

Although the use of epidural opioids alone has been disappointing, satisfactory pain relief following a combination of fentanyl 50 µg with clonidine 120 µg demonstrated that by the avoidance of local anaesthetics by the epidural route, it is possible to preserve motor function capacity.[68]

## Caesarean section

Although caesarean section (CS) is commonly regarded as an adverse obstetric outcome parameter, there seems to be an increasingly common request by informed women for elective CS without medical indication.[69] The most important reasons are fear of labour pain, emergency CS, perineal or urorectal damage, sexual dysfunction and the desire to have a planned delivery. Elective CS is more likely to be performed under regional anaesthesia. Its opponents often exaggerate the increased costs but there are also increased neonatal and maternal mortality and morbidity.

Caesarean section, regardless of its indication, is never without risks. Hypotension caused by neuraxial techniques cannot be avoided completely. Although it was shown that prehydration with 1000 ml of crystalloids does not influence the severity or incidence of hypotension, colloids,[70,71] in particular hydroxyethyl starch, may be more effective in decreasing the risk of spinally induced hypotension.[72,73] Low-dose spinal anaesthesia has been facilitated by the addition of opioids. Sufentanil 2.5 µg has been found to be the most optimal dose when added to bupivacaine.[74] In the CSE technique, bupivacaine 5–7.5 mg may be sufficient as the initial spinal dose which can be supplemented by epidural fine-tuning to adjust the level of the block to the desired dermatomal level.[73,75] Whereas in high-dose spinal anaesthesia it was not possible to show any difference between the effects of plain or hyperbaric bupivacaine,[76,77] in lower doses a hyperbaric solution may be preferable.[78]

Other caesarean section-related problems such as deep vein thrombosis, infection, and postoperative pain may be reduced by proper prophylactic measurements. The use of low molecular weight heparins, decreasing platelet counts in the HELLP syndrome and prevention of eclampsia with low-dose acetylsalicylic acid are three major concerns for anaesthetists involved in obstetric anaesthesia. It remains to be demonstrated whether single-dose spinal anaesthesia is safer for these patients.

For postoperative analgesia a single intrathecal morphine dose as small as 100 µg has been shown to offer safe and excellent pain relief during the first 24 hours, without further prolongation or improvement by increasing that dose.[79,80]

# Conclusion

In the last 10 years, developments in labour analgesia techniques have aimed at improving maternal and neonatal safety, obstetric outcome, maternal satisfaction, and comfort. Large double-blind randomised studies are required to provide final evidence with respect to their effect upon outcome and recent studies reveal that factors other than neuraxial analgesia should perhaps be blamed when natural delivery turns into instrumentational and operative delivery. Intrathecal pain relief and the usefulness of ropivacaine and the S(–)-enantiomer of bupivacaine in particular require further clinical investigations to enable more precise fine-tuning of obstetric anaesthesia/analgesia. In both vaginal and operative delivery, there is a noticeable trend towards the use of mixtures of lower and lower concentrations and doses of analgesic drugs.

1 Thorp JA, Hu DH, Albin R et al. The effect of intrapartum epidural analgesia on nulliparous labor: a randomized, controlled, prospective trial. Am J Obstet Gynecol 1993;**169**:851–8.

2 Chestnut DH, Vincent RD, McGrath JM, Choi WW, Bates JN. Does early administration of epidural analgesia affect obstetric outcome in nulliparous women who are receiving intravenous oxytocin? Anesthesiology 1994;**80**:1193–200.

3 Chestnut DH, McGrath JM, Vincent R et al. Does early administration of epidural analgesia affect obstetric outcome in nulliparous women who are in spontaneous labor? Anesthesiology 1994;**80**:1201–8.

4 Ramin SM, Gambling DR, Lucas MJ, Sharma SK, Sidawi JE, Leveno KJ. Randomized trial of epidural versus intravenous analgesia during labor. Obstet Gynecol 1995;**86**:783–9.

5 Sharma SK, Sidawi JE, Ramin SM, Lucas MJ, Leveno KJ, Cunningham FG. Cesarean delivery: a randomized trial of epidural versus patient-controlled meperidine analgesia during labor. Anesthesiology 1997;**87**:487–94.

6 Lieberman E, Lang JM, Frigoletto F, Richardson DK, Ringer SA, Cohen A. Epidural analgesia, intrapartum fever, and neonatal sepsis evaluation. Pediatrics 1997;**99**:415–19.

7 Lieberman E, Cohen A, Lang J, Frigoletto F, Goetzl L. Maternal intrapartum temperature elevation as a risk factor for cesarean delivery and assisted vaginal delivery. Am J Public Health 1999;**89**:506–10.

8 Philip J, Alexander J, Sharma SK, Leveno KJ , McIntire DD, Wiley J. Epidural analgesia during labor and maternal fever. Anesthesiology 1999;**90**:1271–5.

9 Vertommen J, Vandermeulen E, van Aken H et al. The effects of the addition of sufentanil to 0.125% bupivacaine on the quality of analgesia during labor and the incidence of instrumental deliveries. Anesthesiology 1991;**74**:809–14.

10 Olofsson C, Ekblom A, Ekman-Ordeberg G, Irested L. Obstetric outcome following epidural analgesia with bupivacaine-adrenaline 0.25% or bupivacaine 0.125% with sufentanil – a prospective randomized controlled study in 1000 parturients. Acta Anaesthesiol Scand 1998;**42**:284–92.

11 Vertommen JD, Lemmens E, van Aken H. Comparison of the addition of three

different doses of sufentanil to bupivacaine 0.12% given epidurally during labour. *Anaesthesia* 1994;**49**:678–81.

12 Loftus JR, Hill H, Cohen SE. Placental transfer and neonatal effects of epidural sufentanil and fentanyl administration with bupivacaine with bupivacaine during labor. *Anesthesiology* 1995;**83**:300–8.

13 Claes B, Soetens M, van Zundert A, Datta S. Clonidine added to bupivacaine-epinephrine-sufentanil improves analgesia during childbirth. *Reg Anesth Pain Med* 1998;**23**:540–7.

14 Gambling DR, McMorland GH, Yu P, Laszlo C. Comparison of patient-controlled epidural analgesia and conventional intermittent top-up injections during labor. *Anesth Analg* 1990;**70**:256–61.

15 Purdie J, Reid J, Thornburn J, Asbury AJ. Continuous extradural analgesia: comparison of midwife top-ups, continuous infusions and patient controlled administration. *Br J Anaesth* 1992;**68**:580–4.

16 Collis RE, Plaat FS, Morgan BM. Comparison of midwife top-ups, continuous infusion and patient-controlled epidural analgesia for maintaining mobility after a low-dose combined spinal-epidural. *Br J Anaesth* 1999;**82**:233–6.

17 Kumar AA, Vertommen JD, van Aken H. Patient-controlled epidural analgesia during labor using 0.125% bupivacaine and sufentanil. *Anesth Analg* 1993;**76**:S198.

18 Ferrante FM, Rosinia FA, Gordon C, Datta S. The role of continuous background infusions in patient-controlled epidural analgesia for labor and delivery. *Anesth Analg* 1994;**79**:80–4.

19 Vercauteren M, Coppejans H, ten Broecke PW, van Steenberge A, Adriaensen H. Epidural sufentanil for postoperative patient-controlled analgesia (PCA) with or without background infusion: a double-blind comparison. *Anesth Analg* 1995;**80**:76–80.

20 Ferrante FM. 0.0625% bupivacaine with 0.0002% fentanyl via patient-controlled epidural analgesia for pain of labor and delivery. *Clin J Pain* 1995;**11**:121–6.

21 Writer WD, Stienstra R, Eddleston JM *et al.* Neonatal outcome and mode of delivery after epidural analgesia for labour with ropivacaine and bupivacaine: a prospective meta-analysis. *Br J Anaesth* 1998;**81**:713–17.

22 Owen MD, d'Angelo R, Gerancher J *et al.* 0.125% ropivacaine is similar to 0.125% bupivacaine for labor analgesia using patient-controlled epidural infusion. *Anesth Analg* 1998;**86**:527–31.

23 Gautier PE, de Kock M, van Steenberge A, Miclot D, Fanard L, Hody J. Bupivacaine 0.125% or ropivacaine 0.125% with sufentanil for obstetrical analgesia. *Anesthesiology* 1998;**90**:772–8.

24 Capogna G, Celleno D, Fusco P, Lyons G, Columb M. Relative potencies of bupivacaine and ropivacaine for analgesia in labour. *Br J Anaesth* 1999;**82**:371–3.

25 Polley LS, Columb MO, Naughton NN, Wagner D, van de Ven CJ. Relative analgesic potencies of ropivacaine and bupivacaine for epidural analgesia for labor: implications for therapeutic indexes. *Anesthesiology* 1999;**90**:944–50.

26 Viscomi CM, Rathmell JP, Pace NL. Duration of intrathecal analgesia: early versus advanced labor. *Anesth Analg* 1997;**84**:1108–12.

27 Gautier PE, Debry F, Fanard L. Ambulatory combined spinal-epidural analgesia for labor. *Reg Anesth* 1997;**22**:143–7.

28 Campbell DC, Banner R, Crone L-A, Gore-Hickman W, Yip RW. Addition of

epinephrine to intrathecal bupivacaine and sufentanil for ambulatory labor analgesia. *Anesthesiology* 1997;**86**:525–31.

29 Gautier PE, de Kock M, Fanard L, van Steenberge A, Hody JL. Intrathecal clonidine combined with sufentanil for labor analgesia. *Anesthesiology* 1998;**88**:651–6.

30 Herman NL, Calicott R, van Decar TK, Conlin G, Tilton J. Determination of the dose-response relationship for intrathecal sufentanil in laboring patients. *Anesth Analg* 1997;**84**:1256–61.

31 Arkoosh V, Copper M, Norris MC *et al*. Intrathecal sufentanil dose response in nulliparous patients. *Anesthesiology* 1998;**89**:364–70.

32 Vercauteren M, Bettens K, van Springel G, Schols G, van Zundert J. Intrathecal labor analgesia: can we use the same mixture as is used epidurally? *Int J Obst Anesth* 1997;**6**:242–6.

33 Sia AT, Chong JL, Chiu JW. Combination of intrathecal sufentanil 10 µg and bupivacaine 2.5 mg for labor analgesia: is half the dose enough ? *Anesth Analg* 1999;**88**:362–6.

34 Hays RL, Palmer CM. Respiratory depression after intrathecal sufentanil during labor. *Anesthesiology* 1994;**81**:511–12.

35 Greenhalgh CA. Respiratory arrest in a parturient following intrathecal injection of sufentanil and bupivacaine. *Anaesthesia* 1996;**51**:173–5.

36 Hamilton CL, Cohen SE. High sensory block after intrathecal sufentanil for labor analgesia. *Anesthesiology* 1995;**83**:1118–21.

37 Ferouz F, Norris MC, Leighton BL. Risk of respiratory arrest after intrathecal sufentanil. *Anesth Analg* 1997;**85**:1088–90.

38 Norris MC, Grieco WM, Borkowski M *et al*. Complications of labor analgesia: epidural versus combined spinal epidural techniques. *Anesth Analg* 1994;**79**:529–37.

39 Wee M. Meningitis after combined spinal-extradural anaesthesia in obstetrics. *Br J Anaesth* 1995;**74**:351.

40 Harding SA, Collis RE, Morgan BM. Meningitis after combined spinal extradural anaesthesia in obstetrics. *Br J Anaesth* 1994;**73**:545–7.

41 Leighton BL, Arkoosh VA, Huffnagle S, Huffnagle HJ, Kinsella SM, Norris MC. The dermatomal spread of epidural analgesia with and without prior intrathecal sufentanil. *Anesth Analg* 1996;**83**:526–9.

42 Clarke VT, Smiley RM, Finster M. Uterine hyperactivity after intrathecal injection of fentanyl for analgesia during labor: a cause of fetal bradycardia? *Anesthesiology* 1994;**81**:1083.

43 Friedlander JD, Fox HE, Cain CF, Dominguez CL, Smiley RM. Fetal bradycardia and uterine hyperactivity following subarachnoid administration of fentanyl during labor. *Reg Anesth* 1997;**22**:378–81.

44 Herbstman C, Zaidan J, O'Neil L, Newman L. Fetal bradycardia and uterine hypertonicity after intrathecal fentanyl in laboring women. *Anesthesiology* 1997;**87**:A873.

45 Gambling DR, Sharma SK, Ramin SM *et al*. A randomized study of combined spinal-epidural analgesia versus intravenous meperidine during labor: impact on cesarean delivery rate. *Anesthesiology* 1998;**89**:1336–44.

46 Nielsen PE, Erickson JR, Abouleish EI, Periatt S, Sheppard C. Fetal heart rate changes after intrathecal sufentanil or epidural bupivacaine for labor analgesia: incidence and clinical significance. *Anesth Analg* 1996;**83**:742–6.

47 Nageotte MP, Larson D, Rumney PJ, Sidhu M, Hollenbach K. Epidural anal-

gesia compared with combined spinal-epidural analgesia during labor in nulliparous women. *N Engl J Med* 1997;**337**:1715–19.

48  Fogel S, Daftary AR, Norris M, Dalman HM, Holtmann B. The incidence of clinically important fetal heart rate abnormalities with combined spinal/epidural vs epidural anesthesia for labor. *Reg Anesth Pain Med* 1999;**24**:S75.

49  Caldwell LE, Rosen MA, Shnider SM. Subarachnoid morphine and fentanyl for labor analgesia: efficacy and adverse effects. *Reg Anesth* 1994;**19**:2–8.

50  Collis RE, Davies DWL, Aveling W. Randomised comparison of combined spinal-epidural and standard epidural analgesia in labour. *Lancet* 1995;**345**:1413–16.

51  D'Angelo R, Anderson MT, Philip J, Eisenach JC. Intrathecal sufentanil compared to epidural bupivacaine for labor analgesia. *Anesthesiology* 1994;**80**:1209–15.

52  Kartawiadi SL, Vercauteren MP, van Steenberge AL, Adriaensen H. Spinal analgesia during labor with low dose bupivacaine, sufentanil and epinephrine: a comparison with epidural analgesia. *Reg Anesth* 1996;**21**:191–6.

53  Price C, Lafreniere L, Brosnan C, Findley I. Regional analgesia in early active labour: combined spinal epidural vs epidural. *Anaesthesia* 1998;**53**:951–5.

54  May AE, Elton CD. Ambulatory extradural analgesia in labour reduces risk of caesarean section. *Br J Anaesth* 1996;**77**:692–3.

55  Levin A, Datta S, Camann WR. Intrathecal ropivacaine for labor analgesia: a comparison with bupivacaine. *Anesth Analg* 1998;**87**:624–7.

56  Wali A, Suresh MS, Vadhera RB. Determination of dose response for intrathecal ropivacaine in laboring parturients (SOAP congress abstract). *Anesthesiology* 1999;**90**:A71.

57  Abboud T, Zhu J, Sharp R, LaGrange C, Rosa C, Kassells B. The efficacy of intrathecal injection of sufentanil using a microspinal catheter for labor analgesia. *Acta Anaesthesiol Scand* 1996;**40**:210–16.

58  Arkoosh VA, Pammer CM, van Maren GA *et al.* Continuous intrathecal labor analgesia: safety and efficacy. *Anesthesiology* 1998;**88**:A8.

59  Al-Mufti R, Morey R, Shennan A, Morgan B. Blood pressure and fetal heart rate changes with patient-controlled combined spinal-epidural analgesia while ambulating in labour. *Br J Obstet Gynaecol* 1997;**102**:192–7.

60  Bloom SL, McIntire DD, Kelly MA *et al.* Lack of effect of walking on labor and delivery. *N Engl J Med* 1998;**339**:76–9.

61  Collis RE, Harding SA, Morgan BM. Effect of maternal ambulation on labour with low-dose combined spinal-epidural analgesia. *Anaesthesia* 1999;**54**:535–9.

62  Buggy D, Hughes N, Gardiner J. Posterior column sensory impairment during ambulatory extradural analgesia in labour. *Br J Anaesth* 1994;**73**:540–2.

63  Abrahams M, Higgins P, Whyte P, Breen P, Muttu S, Gardiner J. Intact proprioception and control of labour pain during epidural analgesia. *Acta Anaesthesiol Scand* 1999;**43**:46–50.

64  Parry MG, Fernando R, Bawa GP, Poulton BB. Dorsal column function after epidural and spinal blockade: implications for the safety of walking following low-dose regional analgesia for labour. *Anaesthesia* 1998;**53**:382–7.

65  Breen TW, Shapiro T, Glaa B, Forster-Payne D, Oriol NE. Epidural anesthesia for labor in an ambulatory patient. *Anesth Analg* 1993;**77**:919–24.

66  James KS, McGrady E, Quasim I, Patrick A. Comparison of epidural bolus administration of 0.25% bupivacaine and 0.1% bupivacaine with 0.0002% fentanyl for analgesia during labour. *Br J Anaesth* 1998;**81**:507–10.

67  Zwack R, Campbell DC, Sawatzky K, Crone LA, Yip RW. Ambulatory labor epidural analgesia: bupivacaine vs ropivacaine (SOAP congress abstract). *Anesthesiology* 1999;**90**:A89.

68  Buggy DJ, MacDowell C. Extradural analgesia with clonidine and fentanyl compared with 0.25% bupivacaine in the frst stage of labour. *Br J Anaesth* 1996;**76**:319–21.

69  Erskine KJ, McGrady E. It is every woman's right to choose to be delivered by elective caesarean section. *Int J Obstet Anesth* 1999;**9**:43–8.

70  Jackson R, Reid JA, Thorburn J. Volume preloading is not essential to prevent spinal-induced hypotension at Caesarean section. *Br J Anaesth* 1995;**75**:262–5.

71  Husaini SW, Russell IF. Volume preload: lack of effect in the prevention of spinal-induced hypotension at Caesarean section. *Int J Obstet Anesth* 1998;**7**:76–81.

72  Riley ET, Cohen SE, Rubenstein AJ, Flanagan B. Prevention of hypotension after spinal anestheia for cesarean section: six percent hetastarch versus lactated Ringer's solution. *Anesth Analg* 1995;**81**:838–42.

73  Vercauteren M, Hoffmann V, Coppejans H, van Steenberge A, Adriaensen H. Hydroxyethylstarch compared with modified gelatin as volume preload before spinal anaesthesia for Caesarean section. *Br J Anaesth* 1996;**76**:731–3.

74  Dahlgren G, Hulstrand C, Jakobsson J, Norman M, Eriksson EW, Martin H. Intrathecal sufentanil, fentanyl or placebo added to bupivacaine for cesarean section. *Anesth Analg* 1997;**85**:1288–93.

75  Fan SZ, Susetio L, Wanh YP, Cheng YJ, Liu CC. Low dose of intrathecal hyperbaric bupivacaine combined with epidural lidocaine for cesarean section – a balanced block technique: looking for the adequate spinal dose. *Anesth Analg* 1994;**78**:474–7.

76  Russell IF, Holmqvist EL. Subarachnoid analgesia for Caesarean section: a double-blind comparison of plain and hyperbaric bupivacaine 0.5%. *Br J Anaesth* 1989;**59**:347–53.

77  Richardson MG, Collins HV, Wissler RN. Intrathecal hypobaric versus hyperbaric bupivacaine with morphine for cesarean section. *Anesth Analg* 1998;**87**:336–40.

78  Vercauteren M, Coppejans H, Hoffmann V, Saldien V, Adriaensen H. Small-dose hyperbaric versus plain bupivacaine during spinal anesthesia for cesarean section. *Anesth Analg* 1998;**86**:989–93.

79  Palmer CM, Emerson S, Volgoropolous D, Alves D. Dose-response relationship of intrathecal morphine for postcesarean analgesia. *Anesthesiology* 1999;**90**:437–44.

80  Milner AR, Bogod DG, Harwood RJ. Intrathecal administration of morphine for elective Caesarean section: a comparison between 0.1 mg and 0.2 mg. *Anaesthesia* 1996;**51**:871–3.

# 8: Controversies in clinical practice of regional anaesthesia

MARKUS C SCHNEIDER, KARL F HAMPL, STEEN PETERSEN-FELIX

## Introduction

The beauty of regional anaesthesia has its roots in the mixture of challenges requiring manual skill in combination with a thorough understanding of pharmacology and anatomy. Regional anaesthesia represents a field of practice where art and science meet, tradition and progress compete, and personal experience and common practice collide. This particular blend provides the forum for heated arguments about views often based on apocryphal anecdotes rather than evidence.

Policies of regional anaesthesia are shaped by long-standing routine and experience; thus, attempts at changing practice patterns tend to meet with resistance. This chapter focuses on three topics which have caused some concern in the recent past and are still triggering debates. These topics are (1) the technique of choice for axillary brachial plexus block, (2) the epidural test dose, and (3) transient neurological symptoms after spinal anaesthesia. Obviously, we do not intend to resolve these controversies but we will provide an update of information based on well-conducted studies in order to encourage sound clinical practice. Any improvement in standards of care will finally accrue to patient outcome.

## Axillary brachial plexus block: is there a technique of choice?

### Outcome studies

There are multiple anatomical sites from which to approach the brachial plexus for regional anaesthetics in the context of surgery involving the upper extremity. Obviously, the current popularity of the axillary brachial plexus block (ABPB) is based in part on its excellent safety record, which appears superior to that of alternative techniques such as the infraclavicular, supraclavicular or interscalene approach. Such an assumption is supported by figures on local anaesthetic-induced systemic toxicity resulting in seizures.[1] Among 25 697 subjects surveyed between 1985 and 1992, 7532 were administered a brachial plexus block using either the axillary (n = 6620), interscalene (n = 659) or supraclavicular (n = 253) approach. In total, 15 patients developed seizures. There were significant differences in seizure frequencies for axillary (0.12%; 95% CI 0.05–0.24), supraclavicular (0.79%; 95% CI 0.1–2.36), and interscalene blocks (0.76%; 95% CI 0.25–1.77). In addition, complications resulting from inadvertent pleural, epidural or intrathecal punctures are less likely as ABPB is performed at a safe distance from both the lung and the vertebral column.

In contrast to the low-risk profile of ABPB in terms of systemic and local complications, there is some controversy regarding its potential for neurovascular injury. Whatever the incidence of permanent neurological sequelae following brachial plexus blocks, the fear of potential neural trauma caused by the injection needle has been and still is the focus of much attention.[2-6] Consequently, the technique used for identifying the brachial plexus rather than the injection site came under close scrutiny.

In 1979, 10 cases of neuropathy attributable to anaesthesia were reported in a prospective study involving 533 patients.[2] Eight of these cases were found in patients in whom paraesthesiae were elicited deliberately (n = 290) but only in two cases in whom the axillary plexus was located without actively eliciting paraesthesiase (n = 243). The difference in the incidence of neuropathy (2.8% versus 0.8%) was not statistically different. However, the author concluded that this result would point in favour of the non-paraesthesia group, thereby disregarding important limitations imposed by study design such as lack of randomisation, an incidence of unintentional paresthaesiase in 40% of patients in the non-paraesthesia group, inconsistencies in drug administration, and the use of standard long-bevel needles.

Subsequent studies have reexamined the issue of nerve injury associated with peripheral nerve blocks. In a prospective study including 854 consecutive patients in the majority of whom at least one paraesthesia had been elicited during the procedure, the overall incidence of postblock neuropathy was only 0.36%.[7] In a broad-scale prospective survey of serious complications related to regional anaesthesia, only four cases of neurological injury were reported after 21 278 peripheral nerve blocks; in all nerve blocks, the procedure was associated with paraesthesia during puncture.[8] This corresponds to an incidence of only 1.9 cases per 10 000 procedures (95% CI

0.5–4.8). Obviously, at such a low frequency, very large numbers of patients are required to identify critical events leading to an adverse outcome. Otherwise, the possibility of a bias is introduced because studies involving too few patients may miss the necessary power to discriminate between causal and coincidental outcomes. In another prospective study involving 1000 consecutive outpatients, the incidence of sensory paraesthesiae attributable to ABPB was very low (0.2%) and full recovery was observed within one month.[9]

The relative safety of ABPB was corroborated by another prospective observational study involving 242 patients.[10] On the first postoperative day, 19% complained of paraesthesiae that persisted in 5% for two weeks and disappeared in all but one case by one month. Of note, none of the newly acquired postoperative neuropathies was related to the anaesthetic technique, as both arterial puncture (n = 217) and paraesthesiae (n = 103) were used for localisation.

An analysis of data from the American Society of Anesthesiologists Closed Claims Project shows that among a total of 4183 cases between 1974 and 1995, 670 claims (16%) were filed for anaesthesia-related nerve injuries.[11] With a proportion of 20%, the brachial plexus was the second most common site of injury after the ulnar nerve (28%). Only in 32% of brachial plexus injuries (n = 83) could the mechanism of injury be identified. Among the 13 brachial plexus injuries attributed to regional anaesthesia following axillary (n = 8), interscalene (n = 4) or supraclavicular (n = 1) blocks, paraesthesiae were specifically noted in four cases of ABPB. However, paraesthesiae were not present in three ABPB resulting in ulnar nerve injury. Conversely, paraesthesiae occurred in one of two cases of median nerve (n = 5) or radial nerve injuries (n = 3) related to ABPB.

Despite multiple aetiologies of neural damage, regional anaesthetic procedures per se often end up being implicated as the most likely damaging event for lack of irrefutable proofs of alternative causes. A retrospective analysis of 1614 ABPB performed over a 10-year period in 607 patients emphasised that among 62 neurological complications only seven (11%) were related to the anaesthetic technique, whereas the majority (89%) resulted from the surgical procedure.[12] In contrast to total surgical tourniquet time, which was associated with an increased risk of neurological complications, neither elicitation of paraesthesiae nor type of needle were significant risk factors for neurological injury. Of note, the risk of persistent paresthesiae was not increased when repeating the block, even within a one-week interval. Neurological complications related to anaesthesia persisted for four (range 0.1–20) weeks whereas complications related to surgery persisted for 12 (range 0.1–364) weeks. Apart from direct damage of neural structures by the needles, vascular injury resulting in arterial spasm or haematoma formation[9] can, in very rare cases, compromise neural function.[13]

117

## Studies evaluating different techniques of ABPB

The following principal methods are used to induce ABPB.

- *The transarterial technique:* a local anaesthetic bolus is injected periarterially on both sides of the axillary artery after a negative blood aspiration test.
- *The paraesthesia technique:* administration of local anaesthetic by single or multiple injections once specific paraesthesiae are elicited by the needle.
- *The perivascular catheter technique:*[14] bolus injection of local anaesthetic via catheter once the neurovascular bundle has been entered ("snap" or "pop" on perforation of its sheath).
- *The nerve stimulator technique:* administration of local anaesthetic by single or multiple injections once one or more of the branches of the brachial plexus are identified by elicitation of specific twitches.

Since the reintroduction of ABPB into clinical practice in the 1960s,[15] each of these techniques has continued to develop independently and find both proponents and opponents. Therefore, current clinical practice may sometimes reflect personal predilection rather than best evidence.

In a prospective study on 100 patients, the reliability of the transarterial approach to the brachial plexus was demonstrated using a standard dose of 50 ml of 1.5% mepivacaine. As there was only one complete block failure, a staggering 99% success rate was obtained.[16] Although no clinical signs of local anaesthetic toxicity were detected, mepivacaine plasma levels peaked at $3.3 \pm 1.3\,\mu g/ml$. This success rate was not duplicated in a similar randomised study using the same mepivacaine dose with adrenaline.[17] In another prospective trial in only 50 patients, block failure after 45 ml of 1% mepivacaine with adrenaline led to general anaesthesia in 16% of patients.[18]

In a randomised study of 59 patients, the use of a nerve stimulator for single-injection ABPB did not improve the success rate (70%) compared with the transarterial (79%) or the single paraesthesia technique (80%).[19] In contrast, only one of 15 patients included in another prospective randomised trial required supplementation of ABPB with the requirement that all four major nerves or the musculocutaneous nerve and another of the main plexus nerves had been blocked.[20]

In a prospective randomised trial, three methods of ABPB were compared in 100 patients.[21] Using a 40 ml volume of 1.5% lignocaine with adrenaline, success rates were not different and ranged from 56% (catheter) to 72% (nerve stimulator) to 82% (paraesthesiae). However, by increasing the number of nerves detected by eliciting paraesthesiae or nerve stimulation from one to three, the success rate was increased to 100%. In this study, the catheter technique did not work in 20% of the cases. Similarly, multiple instead of a single-injection technique using mepivacaine 1% with adrenaline and electrolocation shortened time to readiness for surgery from

38 min to 25 min in 80 patients participating in another double-blind randomised trial.[22] Consequently, requirement for supplemental nerve blocks was significantly decreased from 57% to 7%. The same group performed further double-blind studies comparing the transarterial with the multiple electrical nerve stimulation technique.[23] In the latter group (n = 50), administration of 45 ml of 1% mepivacaine resulted in a significantly higher initial block efficacy (88% versus 61%) and shorter latency of initial block (17 ± 7 versus 25 ± 8 min) than in the transarterial group (n = 50). By using a high-dose regimen consisting of 850 mg mepivacaine with adrenaline in 101 patients, no further clinically significant gain was achieved.[24]

Recently, a multicentre prospective study demonstrated a success rate of 93% in 1650 patients using a multiple injection technique for ABPB.[25] Unintentional paraesthesiae occurred in 17% of patients but only in 17 patients (1%) was transient neurological dysfunction observed during 6 ± 2 weeks. Univariate analysis revealed that a pneumatic tourniquet pressure over 400 mmHg was the only risk factor for the development of neurologic dysfunction (odds ratio 2.9, 95% CI 1.6–5.4) whereas unintentional paraesthesiae were not.

### Recommendations

Currently ABPB practice is characterised by a trend towards the multiple nerve stimulation technique in order to minimise the remote risk of neurovascular harm and to optimise the success rates. In view of extremely low complication rates, personal decision making can be justified, as "Ultimately, the amount of experience with a technique is probably the best indicator of the likelihood of a block succeeding".[14] Such a statement does not necessarily apply to the training situation. Typically, trainees should start by learning the least risky techniques before advancing to more demanding levels of regional anaesthesia. A technique of ABPB that requires placing a sharp needle tip in direct contact with the nerves to be blocked or puncturing the axillary artery introduces some risk of complications and should therefore be discouraged.[4]

## The epidural test dose in obstetric analgesia: do we still need it?

### Background

Over the past decades, obstetric anaesthetic care has evolved from a rather simplistic approach to the unique task of relieving pain during childbirth to more sophisticated policies. Until the advent of regional anaesthetic techniques in this field of practice, the prospects of providing effective analgesia were poor and included methods putting both the mother and her baby at risk. Present-day practice, however, can profit from the vast experience with epidural analgesia gained during almost half a century.

Surprisingly, the controversial files on the usefulness of an epidural test dose in this setting are still far from being closed.[26] The debate was launched by an editorial on cardiac arrests associated with accidental intravascular injection of bupivacaine, following negative aspiration tests, intended for regional anaesthesia.[27] Thereafter, 20 more obstetrical cases, including 16 fatalities, in women receiving bupivacaine for epidural anaesthesia were reported to the Food and Drug Administration of the United States.[28] Obviously, such catastrophes tarnished the safety record of a technique heading for supremacy. Common sense dictates that an epidural catheter be checked for correct position before injection of clinical doses of local anaesthetics to avoid any harm related to incorrect catheter position.

Of course, both real and theoretical concerns continue to exist even though substitution of continuous epidural infusions for intermittent bolus administration, the use of more dilute local anaesthetic solutions, and the availability of multiorifice instead of single end-hole catheters diminish some inherent risks. In the obstetric population, the risk of unintentional epidural vein cannulation is higher than in the non-pregnant population, with frequencies of 5–15% and 2.8% in parturients and in non-pregnant patients, respectively.[29] Similarly, the risk of accidental dural puncture and subarachnoid catheter placement is described as being as high as 0.6–2.7% in the obstetric population.[30] Furthermore, correctly placed epidural catheters may migrate into epidural veins or the subarachnoid space.[31] While unintentional intravascular injection of local anaesthetics results in dose-dependent signs of systemic toxicity, inadvertent subarachnoid injection incurs the risk of total spinal anaesthesia.

## Aspiration test

As the identification of a misplaced epidural catheter is imperative, several safety steps have been recommended and implemented in routine practice. They include a variety of physical and pharmacological tests.

First, by gentle aspiration, the presence of blood (intravascular insertion) or cerebrospinal fluid (subarachnoid misplacement) is excluded. Unfortunately, reliance on aspiration for blood or cerebrospinal fluid alone is hazardous because of false-negative results.[32–36] Using single-hole catheters, routine aspiration of blood often fails to reveal misplacement in an intravascular location. In the literature, frequencies of 33%,[32] 42%,[36] and up to 81%[34] are reported. Such a high rate of false-negative results might be reduced by using multiorifice catheters.[35] Thus, the early popularity of multiorifice catheters in the UK may partially explain why bupivacaine cardiotoxicity has never been considered to be a problem in the UK as it was in the USA. However, in seven of 13 cases when aspiration was impossible, radiological evaluation provided evidence that the multiorifice epidural catheters were positioned intravascularly.[37]

Second, in the case of a negative aspiration test, a drug or a drug mixture is injected to test for specific pharmacological responses suggestive of a subarachnoid or intravenous catheter misplacement.

## Testing for accidental subarachnoid catheter placement

The ongoing controversies about reliable test doses refer to the components necessary to detect intravascular rather than subarachnoid catheter position. In order to reduce the risk of total spinal anaesthesia, the test dose should include only that dosage of local anaesthetic deemed necessary to produce a recognisable and safe level of spinal anaesthesia in the event of accidental dural puncture.[30,33,38] The literature on this issue contains a wealth of different recommendations. In obstetric patients, as little as 30 mg of hyperbaric 1.5% lignocaine and 15 µg adrenaline can suffice to produce a perineal sensory block within two minutes.[33] However, higher doses of lignocaine are commonly used, such as 45 mg isobaric lignocaine with adrenaline,[29,36,39] 60 mg isobaric 2% lignocaine[40] or even 100 mg isobaric 2% lignocaine, the last as a second test dose for parturients developing a tachycardic response to the first adrenaline-containing test dose following a negative aspiration test.[36] As an alternative, a test dose with 12.5 mg bupivacaine and adrenaline is safe.[36]

In a recent double-blind randomised study, the efficacies of adrenaline-containing test doses of 60 mg 2% lignocaine, 7.5 mg 0.25% bupivacaine or 15 mg 0.5% bupivacaine in detecting subarachnoid catheter placement were compared.[41] Despite the limitation that findings in orthopaedic patients are not directly applicable to obstetric subjects, the safety of a 60 mg lignocaine test dose was confirmed as motor block developed in all patients within six minutes following subarachnoid but in none after epidural administration. Similarly, according to another prospective double-blind study involving elderly patients, assessment of motor function by leg raising was 100% sensitive using 45 mg 1.5% lignocaine with adrenaline as a test dose.[42] All patients with truly negative tests were able to raise their legs (negative predictive value 100%). Interestingly, the accuracy of this test was not improved by using additional signs of subarachnoid drug injection such as subjective feeling of warmth or sensory loss by pinprick. In both the aforementioned studies, bupivacaine was less reliable than lignocaine in terms of diagnostic accuracy.[41,42]

In rare cases, an epidural catheter penetrates into the subdural space, the potential space between the dura and the arachnoid. If this occurs, a spinal block typically takes about 20 min to develop once the fragile arachnoid membrane ruptures during a subsequent bolus injection.[30] Identification of this complication is difficult, if not impossible.

## Testing for accidental intravascular catheter placement

A literature search regarding this topic resulted in 267 papers for the period 1980–99. Despite arguments in favour of abandoning the classic test dose for labouring women because of inherent limitations of specificity and sensitivity,[29,36,38] the test dose has not outlived its usefulness.[26] The potential need for an emergency caesarean delivery should certainly not be disregarded in parturients who need epidurals for painful dysfunctional labour. In such a case, large doses of local anaesthetics are required to provide surgical anaesthesia. It is imprudent to jeopardise the safety of parturients by abandoning a diagnostic tool because of its limitations.[43] As the 100% reliable, "perfect" test dose has not yet been defined,[26] a variety of different markers have been studied to examine their clinical suitability and practicability.

### Local anaesthetics

Intravascular injection of a local anaesthetic produces central nervous system symptoms that are dose dependent and manifest as metallic taste, perioral numbness, slurred speech, and tinnitus. For a rapid bolus injection, 1.12 mg/kg of lignocaine was determined as the dose necessary to produce such pretoxic symptoms in 95% of pregnant patients ($ED_{95}$).[40] However, neither the positive nor the negative predictive value of a lignocaine 45–100 mg or a 15 mg bupivacaine test dose has been established in the absence of adrenaline. Therefore, continuous communication with the parturient during the period of test dose administration is important to detect subtle central nervous system alterations.

### Adrenaline

In 1981, 15 µg of adrenaline as a component of the epidural test dose was evaluated for its efficacy in volunteers and sedated non-obstetric patients.[44] In that study, a transient increase in maximum heart rate of almost 30% (approximately 30 beats/min) over control values, accompanied by an increase in systolic blood pressure that occurred within 20–40 seconds and lasted for about three minutes, was observed. But strict criteria for determining a positive test response were not defined. Nevertheless, since then, an admixture of adrenaline to the epidural test dose has become standard practice in surgical patients.

In pregnant women, however, such a clearcut cardiovascular response to adrenaline is missing and marked heart rate variability may mimic positive test results in the absence of a specific drug effect.[45] In the study by Cartwright and co-workers,[45] tachycardia was not only triggered by painful uterine contractions but accelerations in heart rate exceeding 30 beats/min also occurred in 10% of parturients during uterine quiescence. Thus, accepting an increase in heart rate of more than 30 beats/min as a positive test criterion would have introduced a false-positive rate of 12%, including the risk of unnecessary reinsertion of epidural catheters. Furthermore, pregnancy is associated with changes in chronotropic responsiveness to the catecholamines adrenaline[46] and isoproterenol.[47] These changes add to false-negative results and, as a consequence, decrease sensitivity to an adrenaline response.

The limitations of adrenaline as a marker for intravascular injection in labouring women were confirmed in a randomised double-blind study.[46] Using two different (baseline-to-peak and peak-to-peak) criteria as defining a positive heart rate response, only five of 10 versus nine of 10 parturients were correctly identified. Similarly, only four of 10 women who had been injected with intravenous adrenaline developed symptoms (palpitations, headache, anxiety).

These equivocal findings contrast with another publication reporting that in parturients in active labour, an epidural test dose containing 10 or 15 μg of adrenaline was 100% sensitive in detecting intravascular injection.[39] Using a baseline-to-peak criterion of an increase exceeding 10 beats/min within one minute, a specificity of 73% (27% false positive) was observed. The subsequent observational study from the same institution was accompanied by an editorial[43] that pointed to some inherent limitations of the study.[36] Again, a sensitivity of 100% was attributed to the epidural test dose consisting of 15 μg adrenaline and 45 mg lignocaine. This time, a specificity of 96% was achieved using a sudden increase in heart rate of 10 beats/min as a positive diagnostic criterion. In the event of an equivocal response or if a uterine contraction followed within a minute, the test had to be repeated.

It is important to emphasise that foetal safety with a test dose of adrenaline has only been documented in healthy parturients. When properly administered, there were no deleterious effects to the foetus after an epidural dose of 50 μg of adrenaline.[48]

*Isoproterenol*

Isoproterenol, a pure β-adrenergic agonist, is an alternative to adrenaline and offers some theoretical advantages related to the lack of vasoconstrictive action on the uterine vasculature. Double-blind studies in parturients show that a tachycardic response is produced, allowing identification of intravascular injection in all cases.[49] At the same time, isoproterenol increases uterine blood flow.[50] The neurotoxic potential of isoproterenol has not yet been fully investigated and, therefore, the drug should not be used.[51,52]

*Air*

Injection of 1 ml of air has been used successfully to detect intravascular placement of epidural catheters.[34,53] According to the authors, the Doppler transducer of the foetal heart rate monitor can be used by placing the probe over the lower half of the sternum. We infer high professional skills and trained observer ears from the staggering 100% sensitivity and 98% specificity reported.

*Fentanyl*

The use of 100 µg fentanyl has been suggested in order to verify proper epidural catheter placement.[54] Based on prompt appearance of dizziness, drowsiness, and sedation as key findings, a fentanyl effect was more consistently identified after intravenous than epidural administration in this trial with a sensitivity of 100% and a specificity of 95%.

*Nerve stimulator*

By using a metal wire and a nerve stimulator to produce a motor response by low-power stimulation (1–10 mA) of the epidural catheter in 39 parturients, a positive motor response evidenced by truncal or limb movements was observed in all but one woman and indicated correct catheter position.[55] Even a case of intravascular catheter migration was detected by this method. However, more work is required before recommending its utilisation.

# Spinal local anaesthetic toxicity and transient neurological symptoms: what are the facts?

## Background

Recent reports of neurological injury after spinal anaesthesia revived old fears concerning the neurotoxic potential of local anaesthetics. In particular, the safety of spinal lignocaine came under scrutiny, despite a 50-year record of excellence based on its well-established role in clinical practice.[56]

The debate on neurotoxicity was initially launched by a series of case reports of cauda equina syndrome (CES) following continuous spinal anaesthesia[57,58] or accidental subarachnoid injection of lignocaine during intended epidural anaesthesia.[59-61] These concerns were further enhanced by reports of persistent neurological deficits after single-injection spinal anaesthesia as a direct causal relationship could not be excluded.[62-64] Finally, a huge debate was triggered by reports of minor transient side effects observed after uneventful spinal anaesthesia.[65-84] These side effects had a typical neurological pattern of distribution but their nature has not yet been clarified. The intriguing unanswered question was whether these transient neurological symptoms (TNSs), which were characterised by pain and/or dysaesthesia in the buttocks or lower extremities, share a common mechanism with CES. However, the possibility of a common pathophysiological mechanism cannot be discounted with certainty even if the clinical characteristics of CES and TNSs are different. This may explain the continuing enthusiasm of many journals for publishing editorial comments and recommendations as to whether the use of lignocaine for spinal anaesthesia should be continued.[85–90]

## Spinal local anaesthetic toxicity

In 1991, four cases of persistent sacral nerve root deficits diagnosed as CES were observed after continuous spinal anaesthesia.[57] They were attributed to an overdose of local anaesthetic (lignocaine in three cases, amethocaine in one case) and poor mixing of the hyperbaric local anaesthetic solution within the cerebrospinal fluid (CSF), resulting in locally toxic concentrations. This hypothesis was supported by subsequent studies using spinal glass models of the subarachnoid space.[91–93] In response to a cluster of similar reports,[58] spinal microcatheters were withdrawn from the US market to avoid additional catastrophic outcomes.[94] Moreover, three years later the Food and Drug Administration recommended that the package insert of 5% lignocaine should be modified to encourage dilution of this local anaesthetic with an equal volume of CSF prior to spinal application. Thus, exposure of nerve roots to high concentrations of lignocaine would be prevented.

Despite marked changes in spinal anaesthesia policies for fear of causing persistent neurological sequelae, these strategies were bound to fail when accidental dural puncture occurred during intended epidural anaesthesia. Three more cases of CES were subsequently reported, all of them after inadvertent subarachnoid administration of 2% lignocaine.[95–97]

Consideration of the maximum safe dose used for spinal anaesthesia is essential when assessing the neurotoxic potential of local anaesthetics. Differences in local anaesthetic potencies should be taken into account when developing dose recommendations for single as well as repeat injections in the event of block failure. Repeat injections, however, are potentially unsafe even though they may be common practice. Specifically, it was suggested that inadequate sensory block often results from maldistribution of the anaesthetic within the CSF.[98] Therefore, repeat injection might result in neurotoxic concentrations. This concern is supported by a recent case of CES that is possibly attributable to maldistribution and repeat injection of 5% lignocaine.[64] Sometimes, albeit rarely, persistent neurological deficits are observed in patients in whom spinal anaesthesia was performed using recommended doses of a local anaesthetic – a disconcerting finding.[62–64]

## Transient neurological symptoms

In 1993, four patients with TNSs were observed after uneventful spinal anaesthesia with hyperbaric 5% lignocaine.[65] Numerous similar cases in association with hyperbaric 5% lignocaine were subsequently reported.[66,72,74,99–101] Data from non-randomised[68,69,79] and randomised[70,71,81,102] clinical studies support the concept that these symptoms arise from an effect of the local anaesthetic and indicate that TNSs are more common with lignocaine than with other local anaesthetics and relatively uncommon with bupivacaine.

An epidemiologic analysis of factors that increase the incidence of TNSs revealed that lithotomy position and outpatient status are the most significant risk factors in patients who receive lignocaine for spinal anaesthesia.[79] In comparison with bupivacaine and amethocaine, lignocaine increased the risk for TNSs by a factor of 5.1 (95% CI 2.5–10.2) and 3.2 (95% CI 1.04–9.84), respectively. Data from this large-scale epidemiologic, multi-centre study involving 1863 patients show that the lithotomy position increased the relative risk for TNSs by a factor of 2.6 (95% CI 1.5–4.5) compared with other positions. Outpatient status, on the other hand, enhanced the risk for TNSs by a factor of 3.6 (95% CI 1.9–6.8), while obesity was of borderline significance with a relative risk of 1.6 (95% CI 1.0–2.5). Importantly, other factors believed to be significantly associated with TNSs, such as needle type, history of back pain, age, and sex, were excluded as risk factors.

Below, studies are summarised that evaluate the importance of potential risk factors for the occurrence of TNSs. Data from two randomised studies suggest that the osmolarity[70] and the concentration of glucose[70,71] do not affect the incidence of TNSs following lignocaine spinal anaesthesia. Data from two other prospective randomised trials indicate that reducing ligno-caine concentration from 5% to 2% does not decrease the risk for TNSs.[71,103] Apparently, there is no safe low "threshold" concentration of lignocaine in terms of avoiding TNSs as TNSs were observed after spinal anaesthesia using 1% plain lignocaine.[82] According to a randomised trial in outpatients undergoing knee arthroscopy, lignocaine concentrations as low as 0.5% were associated with TNSs.[84] Data on the incidence of TNSs after lignocaine spinal anaesthesia conflict, as a broad range of incidences is reported with 0.4%[104] at the low end and 40% at the high end.[103] Some of these discrepancies may be explained by differences in data sampling, patient positioning and, last but not least, diagnostic criteria used to define TNSs. Studies using non-standardised data collection[105] or retrospective data analysis[80] often find lower incidences of TNSs due to underreporting and failure of patients to respond to questionnaires.[80] In addition, studies of patients operated in the lithotomy position or with flexed knees tend to find higher incidences of TNSs[69,71,79,84,103] than those investigating patients in other positions. It is therefore not surprising that a very low incidence of TNSs was found in a recent prospective study of 1045 patients receiving lignocaine spinal anaesthesia for anorectal surgery performed in the prone jackknife position.[104]

*Aetiology*

The aetiology of TNSs after spinal anaesthesia is unknown. Myofascial pain or facet joint irritation have been suggested as possible aetiologies.[106,107] If so, differences in the incidence of TNSs would indicate differences in musculoligamental relaxation induced by different local anaesthetics.[102] However, any assumption that differences in degree of motor block would explain differences in incidences of TNSs after lignocaine and bupivacaine is purely hypothetical and speculative. Moreover, a difference in intensity of motor block may be completely missing.[108] In a prospective study evaluating the incidence of TNSs in 60 patients randomised to receive either spinal anaesthesia with 5% lignocaine or general anaethesia with neuromuscular relaxation, typical TNSs occurred in 27% of patients in the spinal group whereas a single patient in the general anaesthesia group developed such symptoms, albeit only on postoperative day 3, which does not conform with its clinical definition.[109] More importantly, profound neuromuscular relaxation did not contribute to the occurrence of TNSs following general anaesthesia.

## Alternatives to lignocaine

*Bupivacaine* is associated with a significantly decreased risk of postoperative TNSs compared with lignocaine.[69-71,79] However, as a long-acting drug it is far from being a good alternative to lignocaine and is not suitable for short surgical procedures, particularly in ambulatory patients.

*Mepivacaine* and lignocaine are similar in duration of action. There have been a few case reports of patients with TNSs after mepivacaine spinal anaesthesia.[110,111] However, the results of prospective studies comparing the incidences of TNSs associated with lignocaine and mepivacaine are limited and conflicting. In a prospective randomised study of ambulatory patients undergoing knee arthroscopy, 2% mepivacaine was not associated with TNSs whereas TNSs occurred in 22% of patients receiving 1.5% lignocaine.[83] In contrast, results from another prospective randomised study suggested an increased risk for TNSs with 4% mepivacaine compared with 0.5% bupivacaine.[112] In a further prospective trial of 90 patients undergoing mainly urological procedures, the incidence of TNSs was 20% for CSF-diluted 5% lignocaine, 37% for 4% mepivacaine, and zero in patients receiving 0.5% bupivacaine.[102]

*Prilocaine* and lignocaine are similar in potency and duration of action. In a previous survey of more than 5000 patients, TNSs were not observed.[113] In a recent randomised study comparing prilocaine with lignocaine in 90 patients undergoing short gynaecological procedures in the lithotomy position, the incidence of TNSs was 32% for 2% lignocaine, 3% for 2% prilocaine, and zero in patients receiving 0.5% bupivacaine.[81] Conversely, according to another study comparing 198 patients undergoing various surgical procedures, there was no statistically significant difference in incidences of TNSs, which were 4.1% in the 5% lignocaine and 1% in the 5% prilocaine group, respectively.[114] However, only 17 patients per study group were operated in the lithotomy position and thus a major risk factor was absent.[79]

*Procaine*, an ester-type local anaesthetic with a short duration of action, is not popular for spinal anaesthesia in Europe. In a recent prospective pilot study evaluating the suitability of 10% procaine in 106 patients, only one individual complained of TNSs.[115] In another recent study, comparing 10% procaine with or without the addition of adrenaline, the incidence of TNSs was 1.7%.[116] However, controlled randomised comparative studies are needed to further evaluate its safety and risk profile as a local anaesthetic, although it is still marketed as a highly concentrated 10% solution for spinal anaesthesia.

## Recommendations

Recent clinical experience has generated concern about the potential neurotoxicity of local anaesthetics currently used for spinal anaesthesia. Surprisingly, lignocaine has been the focus of much attention despite its previous untarnished safety record. For a long time, lignocaine has been considered by many to be the gold standard for spinal anaesthetics of short duration. Review of reports of clincal injury and recent experimental data have led to a number of recommendations to decrease the risk of injury.[57,88,98] They include the administration of the lowest effective local anaesthetic concentration, the observation of a 60 mg ceiling dose for spinal lignocaine, and the avoidance of adrenaline for prolongation of lignocaine spinal anaesthesia.

In addition to rare reports of persistent neurological injury, numerous studies document the common occurrence of TNSs after uneventful single injection of lignocaine for spinal anaesthesia. There is a lot of evidence identifying the lithotomy position and outpatient status as major risk co-factors. Unfortunately, the incidence of TNSs is not reduced by using more dilute lignocaine solutions or lower doses. There are insufficient data on alternative short-acting local anaesthetics to use as substitutes for lignocaine. Further studies are thus needed to establish the suitability and safety of mepivacaine, prilocaine, and procaine when used for spinal anaesthesia. The usefulness and clinical practicality of low doses of a long-acting local anaesthetic such as bupivacaine, which rarely causes TNSs, and perhaps in the future also of levobupivacaine and ropivacaine, for spinal anaesthesia of short duration should also be evaluated.

1 Brown DL, Ransom DM, Hall JA, Leicht CH, Schroeder DR, Offord KP. Regional anesthesia and local anesthetic-induced systemic toxicity: seizure frequency and accompanying cardiovascular changes. *Anesth Analg* 1995;**81**:321–8.

2 Selander D, Edshage S, Wolff T. Paresthesia or no paresthesia? Nerve lesions after axillary blocks. *Acta Anaesthesiol Scand* 1979;**23**:27–33.

3 Selander D. Axillary plexus block: paresthetic or perivascular? [editorial] *Anesthesiology* 1987;**66**:726–8.

4 Chambers WA. Peripheral nerve damage and regional anaesthesia [editorial]. *Br J Anaesth* 1992;**69**:429–30.

5 Moore DC, Mulroy MF, Thompson GE. Peripheral nerve damage and regional anaesthesia [editorial]. *Br J Anaesth* 1994;**73**:435–6.

6 Winnie AP. Does the transarterial technique of axillary block provide a higher success rate and a lower complication rate than a paresthesia technique? *Reg Anesth* 1995;**20**:482–5.

7 Winchell SW, Wolfe R. The incidence of neuropathy following upper extremity nerve blocks. *Reg Anesth* 1985;**10**:12–15.

8 Auroy Y, Narchi P, Messiah A, Litt L, Rouvier B, Samii K. Serious complications related to regional anesthesia. Results of a prospective survey in France. *Anesthesiology* 1997;**87**:479–86.

9 Stan TC, Krantz MA, Solomon DL, Poulos JG, Chaouki K. The incidence of neurovascular complications following axillary brachial plexus block using a transarterial approach. A prospective study of 1,000 consecutive patients. *Reg Anesth* 1995;**20**:486–92.

10 Urban MK, Urquhart B. Evaluation of brachial plexus anesthesia for upper extremity surgery. *Reg Anesth* 1994;**19**:175–82.

11 Cheney FW, Domino KB, Caplan RA, Posner KL. Nerve injury associated with anesthesia. A closed claims analysis. *Anesthesiology* 1999;**90**:1062–9.

12 Horlocker TT, Kufner RP, Bishop AT, Maxson PM, Schroeder DR. The risk of persistent paresthesia is not increased with repeated axillary block. *Anesth Analg* 1999;**88**:382–7.

13 Ben-David B, Stahl S. Axillary block complicated by hematoma and radial nerve injury. *Reg Anesth Pain Med* 1999;**24**:264–6.

14 Partridge BL, Kath J, Benirschke K. Functional anatomy of the brachial plexus sheath: implications for anesthesia. *Anesthesiology* 1987;**66**:743–7.

15 Burnham PJ. Simple regional nerve blocks for surgery for the hand and forearm. *JAMA* 1959;**169**:941–3.

16 Cockings E, Moore PL, Lewis RC. Transarterial brachial plexus blockade using high doses of 1.5% mepivacaine. *Reg Anesth* 1987;**12**:159–64.

17 Hickey R, Hoffmann J, Tingle LJ, Rogers JN, Ramamurthy S. Comparison of the clinical efficacy of three perivascular techniques for axillary brachial plexus block. *Reg Anesth* 1993;**18**:335–8.

18 Pere P, Pitkänen M, Tuominen M, Edgren J, Rosenberg PH. Clinical and radiological comparison of perivascular and transarterial techniques of axillary brachial plexus block. *Br J Anaesth* 1993;**70**:276–9.

19 Goldberg ME, Gregg C, Larijani GE, Norris MC, Marr AT, Seltzer JL. A comparison of three methods of axillary approach to brachial plexus blockade for upper extremity surgery. *Anesthesiology* 1987;**66**:814–16.

20 Lavoie J, Martin R, Tétrault J-P, Côté DJ, Colas MJ. Axillary plexus block using a peripheral nerve stimulator: single or multiple injections. *Can J Anaesth* 1992;**39**:583–6.

21 Baranowski AP, Pither CE. A comparison of three methods of axillary brachial plexus anaesthesia. *Anaesthesia* 1990;**45**:362–5.

22 Koscielniak-Nielsen ZJ, Stans-Pedersen HL, Lippert FK. Readiness for

surgery after axillary block: single or multiple injection techniques. *Eur J Anaesthesiol* 1997;**14**:164–71.

23 Koscielniak-Nielsen ZJ, Hesselberg L, Fejlberg V. Comparison of transarterial and multiple nerve stimulation techniques for an initial axillary block by 45 mL of mepivacaine 1% with adrenaline. *Acta Anaesthesiol Scand* 1998;**42**:570–5.

24 Koscielniak-Nielsen ZJ, Rotbøll Nielsen P, Loumann Nielsen S, Gardi T, Hermann C. Comparison of transarterial and multiple nerve stimulation techniques for axillary block using a high dose of mepivacaine with adrenaline. *Acta Anaesthesiol Scand* 1999;**43**:398–404.

25 Fanelli G, Casati A, Garancini P, Torri G for the Study Group on Regional Anesthesia. Nerve stimulator and multiple injection technique for upper and lower limb blockade: failure rate, patient acceptance, and neurologic complications. *Anesth Analg* 1999;**88**:847–52.

26 Birnbach DJ, Chestnut DH. The epidural test dose in obstetric patients: has it outlived its usefulness? [editorial] *Anesth Analg* 1999;**88**:971–2.

27 Albright GA. Cardiac arrest following regional anesthesia with etidocaine or bupivacaine [editorial]. *Anesthesiology* 1979;**51**:285–7.

28 Santos AC, Pedersen H. Current controversies in obstetric anesthesia. *Anesth Analg* 1994;**78**:753–60.

29 Norris MC, Ferrenbach D, Dalman H *et al*. Does epinephrine improve the diagnostic accuracy of aspiration during labor epidural analgesia? *Anesth Analg* 1999;**88**:1073–6.

30 Richardson MG, Lee AC, Wissler RN. High spinal anesthesia after epidural test dose administration in five obstetric patients. *Reg Anesth* 1996;**21**:119–23.

31 Reynolds F. Epidural catheter migration during labour [letter]. *Anaesthesia* 1988;**43**:69.

32 Kenepp NB, Gutsche BB. Inadvertent intravascular injections during lumbar epidural anesthesia [letter]. *Anesthesiology* 1981;**54**:172–3.

33 Abraham RA, Harris AP, Maxwell LG, Kaplow S. The efficacy of 1.5% lidocaine with 7.5% dextrose and epinephrine as an epidural test dose for obstetrics. *Anesthesiology* 1986;**55**:693–6.

34 Leighton BL, Norris MC, DeSimone CA, Rosko T, Gross JB. The air test as a clinically useful indicator of intravenously placed epidural catheters. *Anesthesiology* 1990;**73**:610–13.

35 Norris MC, Fogel ST, Dalman H, Borrenpohl S, Hoppe W, Riley A. Labor epidural analgesia without an intravascular "test dose". *Anesthesiology* 1998;**88**:1495–501.

36 Colonna-Romano P, Nagaraj L. Tests to evaluate intravenous placement of epidural catheters in laboring women: a prospective clinical study. [Erratum in *Anesth Analg* 1998;**87**:3.] *Anesth Analg* 1998;**86**:985–8.

37 Beck H, Brassow F, Doehn M, Bause H, Dziadzka A, Schulte am Esch J. Epidural catheters of the multi-orifice type: dangers and complications. *Acta Anaesthesiol Scand* 1986;**30**:549–55.

38 Van Zundert A, Vase L, Soetens CA *et al*. Every dose given in epidural analgesia for vaginal delivery can be a test dose. *Anesthesiology* 1987;**67**:436–40.

39 Colonna-Romano P, Lingaraju N, Godfrey SD, Braitman LE. Epidural test dose and intravascular injection in obstetrics: sensitivity, specificity, and lowest effective dose. *Anesth Analg* 1992;**75**:372–6.

40 Strebel S, Frei F, Rosow CE, Drewe J. Central nervous system symptoms after intravenous lignocaine: dose-response during pregnancy. *Eur J Anaesthesiol* 1993;**10**:101–4.

41 Poblete B, van Gessel EF, Gaggero G, Gamulin Z. Efficacy of three test doses to detect epidural catheter misplacement. *Can J Anaesth* 1999;**46**:34–9.

42 Colonna-Romano P, Padolina R, Lingaraju N, Braitman LE. Diagnostic accuracy of an intrathecal test dose in epidural analgesia. *Can J Anaesth* 1994;**41**:572–4.

43 Mulroy M, Glosten B. The epinephrine test dose in obstetrics: note the limitations. *Anesth Analg* 1998;**86**:923–5.

44 Moore DC, Batra MS. The components of an effective test dose prior to epidural block. *Anesthesiology* 1981;**55**:693–6.

45 Cartwright PD, McCarroll SM, Antzaka C. Maternal heart rate changes with a plain epidural test dose. *Anesthesiology* 1986;**65**:226–8.

46 Leighton BL, Norris MC, Sosis M, Epstein R, Chayen B, Larijani GE. Limitations of epinephrine as a marker of intravascular injection in laboring women. *Anesthesiology* 1987;**66**:688–91.

47 DeSimone CA, Leighton BL, Norris MC, Chayen B, Menduke H. The chronotropic effect of isoproterenol is reduced in term pregnant women. *Anesthesiology* 1988;**69**:626–8.

48 Albright GA, Jouppila R, Hollmén AI, Jouppila P, Vierola H, Koivula A. Epinephrine does not alter human intervillous blood flow during epidural anesthesia. *Anesthesiology* 1981;**54**:131–5.

49 Leighton BL, DeSimone CA, Norris MC, Chayen B. Isoproterenol is an effective marker of intravenous injection in laboring women. *Anesthesiology* 1989;**70**:206–9.

50 Marcus MA, Vertommen JD, van Aken H, Wouters PF, van Assche A, Spitz B. Hemodynamic effects of intravenous isoproterenol versus saline in the parturient. *Anesth Analg* 1997;**84**:1113–16.

51 Marcus MA, Vertommen JD, van Aken H, Wouters PF. Hemodynamic effects of intravenous isoproterenol versus epinephrine in the chronic maternal-fetal sheep preparation. *Anesth Analg* 1996;**82**:1023–6.

52 Norris MC, Arkoosh VA, Knobler R. Maternal and fetal effects of isoproterenol in the gravid ewe. *Anesth Analg* 1997;**85**:389–94.

53 Leighton BL, Gross JB. Air: an effective indicator of intravenously located epidural catheters. *Anesthesiology* 1989;**71**:848–51.

54 Yoshii WY, Miller M, Rottman RL *et al*. Fentanyl for epidural intravascular test dose in obstetrics. [Erratum in *Reg Anesth* 1994;**19**: preceding table of contents. *Reg Anesth* 1993;**18**:296–9.

55 Tsui BS, Gupta S, Finucane B. Determination of epidural catheter placement using nerve stimulation in obstetric patients. *Reg Anesth Pain Med* 1999;**24**:17–23.

56 Phillips OC, Ebner H, Nelson AT, Black MH. Neurologic complications following spinal anesthesia with lidocaine: a prospective review of 10,440 cases. *Anesthesiology* 1969;**30**:284–9.

57 Rigler ML, Drasner K, Krejcie TC *et al*. Cauda equina syndrome after continuous spinal anesthesia. *Anesth Analg* 1991;**72**:275–81.

58 Schell RM, Brauer FS, Cole DS, Applegate RL II. Persistent sacral nerve root deficits after continuous spinal anaesthesia. *Can J Anaesth* 1991;**38**:908–11.

59 Drasner K, Rigler ML, Sessler DI, Stoller ML. Cauda equina syndrome following intended epidural anesthesia. *Anesthesiology* 1992;**77**:582–5.

60 Cheng A. Intended epidural anesthesia as a possible cause of cauda equina syndrome. *Anesth Analg* 1993;**78**:157–9.

61 Lee DS, Bui T, Ferrarese J, Richardson PK. Cauda equina syndrome after incidental total spinal anesthesia with 2% lidocaine. *J Clin Anesth* 1998;**10**:66–9.

62 Gerancher JC. Cauda equina syndrome following a single spinal administration of 5% hyperbaric lidocaine through a 25-gauge Whitacre needle. *Anesthesiology* 1997;**87**:687–9.

63 Auroy Y, Narchi P, Messiah A, Litt L, Rouvier B, Samii K. Serious complications related to regional anesthesia. Results of a prospective survey in France. *Anesthesiology* 1997;**87**:479–86.

64 Loo CC, Irestedt L. Cauda equina syndrome after spinal anaesthesia with hyperbaric 5% lignocaine: a review of six cases of cauda equina syndrome reported to the Swedish Pharmaceutical Insurance 1993–1997. Acta Anaesthesiol Scand 1999;**43**:371–9.

65 Schneider M, Ettlin T, Kaufmann M *et al.* Transient neurologic toxicity after hyperbaric subarachnoid anesthesia with 5% lidocaine. *Anesth Analg* 1993;**76**:1154–7.

66 Sjöström S, Bläss J. Severe pain in both legs after spinal anaesthesia with hyperbaric 5% lignocaine solution. *Anaesthesia* 1994;**49**:700–2.

67 Pinczower GR, Chadwick HS, Woodland R, Lowmiller M. Bilateral leg pain following lidocaine spinal anaesthesia. *Can J Anaesth* 1995;**42**:217–20.

68 Tarkkila P, Huhtala J, Tuominen M. Transient radicular irritation after spinal anaesthesia with hyperbaric 5% lignocaine. *Br J Anaesth* 1995;**74**:328–9.

69 Hampl KF, Schneider MC, Ummenhofer W, Drewe J. Transient neurologic symptoms after spinal anesthesia. *Anesth Analg* 1995;**81**:1148–53.

70 Hampl KF, Schneider MC, Thorin D, Ummenhofer W, Drewe J. Hyperosmolarity does not contribute to transient radicular irritation after spinal anesthesia with hyperbaric 5% lidocaine. *Reg Anesth* 1995;**20**:363–8.

71 Pollock J, Neal J, Stephenson C, Wiley C. Prospective study of the incidence of transient radicular irritation in patients undergoing spinal anesthesia. *Anesthesiology* 1996;**84**:1361–7.

72 Albrecht A, Hogg M, Robinson S. Transient radicular irritation as a complication of spinal anaesthesia with hyperbaric 5% lignocaine. *Anaesth Intens Care* 1996;**24**:508–10.

73 Fenerty J, Sonner J, Sakura S, Drasner K. Transient radicular pain following spinal anesthesia: review of the literature and report of a case involving 2% lidocaine. *Int J Obst Anesth* 1996;**5**:32–5.

74 Rodriguez-Chinchilla R, Rodriguez-Pont A, Pintanel T, Vidal-Lopez F. Bilateral severe pain at L3-4 after spinal anaesthesia with hyperbaric 5% lignocaine. *Br J Anaesth* 1996;**76**:328–9.

75 Salmela L, Aromaa U, Cozanitis DA. Leg and back pain after spinal anasethesia involving hyperbaric 5% lignocaine. *Anaesthesia* 1996;**51**:391–3.

76 Demeere JL, Naud J-L. Neurological pain after subarachnoid anaesthesia with lidocaine. *Br J Anaesth* 1997;**78**:5–6.

77 Grange C, Bright S, Douglas J. Radicular irritation with 2% lignocaine spinal. *Anaesth Intens Care* 1997;**25**:89–90.

78 Ramasamy D, Eadie R. Transient radicular irritation after spinal anaesthesia with 2% isobaric lignocaine. *Br J Anaesth* 1997;**79**:394–5.

79 Freedman JM, Li DK, Drasner K, Jaskela MC, Larsen B, Wi S. Transient neurologic symptoms after spinal anesthesia: an epidemiologic study of 1,863 patients. *Anesthesiology* 1998;**89**:633–41.

80  Corbey MP, Bach AB. Transient radicular irritation (TRI) after spinal anesthesia in day-care surgery. *Acta Anaesthesiol Scand* 1998;**42**:425–9.

81  Hampl KF, Heinzmann-Wiedmer S, Luginbühl I *et al.* Transient neurologic symptoms after spinal anesthesia: a lower incidence with prilocaine and bupivacaine than with lidocaine. *Anesthesiology* 1998;**88**:629–33.

82  Henderson DJ, Faccenda KA, Morrison LMM. Transient radicular irritation with intrathecal plain lignocaine. *Acta Anaesthesiol Scand* 1998;**42**:376–8.

83  Liguori GA, Zayas VM, Chisholm MF. Transient neurologic symptoms after spinal anesthesia with mepivacaine and lidocaine. *Anesthesiology* 1998;**88**:619–23.

84  Pollock JE, Liu SS, Neal JM, Stephenson CA. Dilution of spinal lidocaine does not alter the incidence of transient neurologic symptoms. *Anesthesiology* 1999;**90**:445–50.

85  De Jong R. Last round for a "heavyweight"? *Anesth Analg* 1994;**78**:3–4.

86  Douglas MJ. Neurotoxicity of lidocaine – does it exist? *Can J Anaesth* 1995;**42**:181–5.

87  Carpenter R. Hyperbaric lidocaine spinal anesthesia: do we need an alternative? *Anesth Analg* 1995;**81**:1125–8.

88  Drasner K. Lidocaine spinal anesthesia. A vanishing therapeutic index? *Anesthesiology* 1997;**87**:469–72.

89  Dahlgren N. Lidocaine toxicity: a technical knock-out below the waist? *Acta Anaesthesiol Scand* 1998;**42**:389–90.

90  Neal JM, Pollock JE. Can scapegoats stand on shifting sands? *Reg Anesth Pain Med* 1998;**23**:533–7.

91  Rigler ML, Drasner K. Distribution of catheter-injected local anesthetic in a model of the subarachnoid space. *Anesthesiology* 1991;**75**:684–92.

92  Ross BK, Coda B, Heath CH. Local anesthetic distribution in a spinal model: a possible mechanism of neurologic injury after continuous spinal anesthesia. *Reg Anesth* 1992;**17**:69–77.

93  Robinson RA, Stewart SF, Myers MR *et al.* In vitro modeling of spinal anesthesia. A digital video image processing technique and its application to catheter characterization. *Anesthesiology* 1994;**81**:1053–60.

94  FDA Safety Alert May 29, 1992. Cauda equina syndrome associated with the use of small-bore catheters in continuous spinal anesthesia.

95  Drasner K, Rigler ML, Sessler DI, Stoller ML. Cauda equina syndrome following intended epidural anesthesia. *Anesthesiology* 1992;**77**:582–5.

96  Cheng A. Intended epidural anesthesia as a possible cause of cauda equina syndrome. *Anesth Analg* 1993;**78**:157–9.

97  Lee DS, Bui T, Ferrarese J, Richardson PK. Cauda equina syndrome after incidental total spinal anesthesia with 2% lidocaine. *J Clin Anesth* 1998;**10**:66–9.

98  Drasner K, Rigler M. Repeat injection after a "failed spinal": at times, a potentially unsafe practice. *Anesthesiology* 1991;**75**:713–14.

99  Snyder R, Hui G, Flugstad P, Viarengo C. More cases of possible neurologic toxicity associated with single subarachnoid injections of 5% hyperbaric lidocaine [letter]. *Anesth Analg* 1994;**78**:411.

100  Newman LM, Iyer NR, Tuman KJ. Transient radicular irritation after hyperbaric lidocaine spinal anesthesia in parturients. *Int J Obst Anesth* 1997;**6**:132–4.

101  Panadero A, Monedero P, Fernandez-Liesa JI, Percaz J, Olavide I, Irribarren MJ. Repeated transient neurologic symptoms after spinal anaesthesia with hyperbaric 5% lidocaine. *Br J Anaesth* 1998;**81**:471–2.

102 Salmela L, Aromaa U. Transient radicular irritation after spinal anesthesia induced with hyperbaric solutions of cerebrospinal fluid-diluted lidocaine 50 mg/ml or mepivacaine 40 mg/ml or bupivacaine 5 mg/ml. *Acta Anaesthesiol Scand* 1998;**42**:765–9.

103 Hampl KF, Schneider MC, Pargger H, Gut M, Drewe J, Drasner K. A similar incidence of transient neurologic symptoms after spinal anesthesia with 2% and 5% lidocaine. *Anesth Analg* 1996;**83**:1051–4.

104 Morisaki H, Masuda J, Kaneko S, Matsushima M, Takeda J. Transient neurologic syndrome in one thousand forty-five patients after 3% lidocaine spinal anesthesia. *Anesth Analg* 1998;**86**:1023–6.

105 Dahlgren N, Törnebrandt K. Neurological complications after spinal anesthesia. A follow-up of 18 000 spinal and epidural anaesthetics performed over three years. *Acta Anaesthesiol Scand* 1995;**39**:872–80.

106 Hartrick CT. Transient radicular irritation – a misnomer? *Anesth Analg* 1997;**84**:1392–3.

107 Naveira FA, Copeland S, Anderson M, Speight K, Rauck R. Transient neurologic toxicity after spinal anesthesia, or is it myofascial pain? Two case reports. *Anesthesiology* 1998;**88**:268–70.

108 Ewart MC, Rubin AP. Subarachnoid block with hyperbaric lignocaine. A comparison with hyperbaric bupivacaine. *Anaesthesia* 1987;**42**:1183–7.

109 Hiller A, Karjalainen K, Balk M, Rosenberg PH. Transient neurological symptoms after spinal anaesthesia with hyperbaric 5% lidocaine or general anaesthesia. *Br J Anaesth* 1999;**82**:575–9.

110 Lynch J, zur Nieden M, Kasper SM, Radbruch L. Transient radicular irritation after spinal anesthesia with hyperbaric 4% mepivacaine. *Anesth Analg* 1997;**85**:872–3.

111 Sia S, Pullano C. Transient radicular irritation after spinal anaesthesia with 2% isobaric mepivacaine. *Br J Anaesth* 1998;**81**:622–4.

112 Hiller A, Rosenberg PH. Transient neurological symptoms after spinal anaesthesia with 4% mepivacaine and 0.5% bupivacaine. *Br J Anaesth* 1997;**79**:301–5.

113 Koenig W, Ruzicic D. Absence of transient radicular irritation after 5000 spinal anaesthetics with prilocaine. *Anaesthesia* 1997;**52**:182–3.

114 Martinez-Bourio R, Arzuaga M, Quintana JM *et al.* Incidence of transient neurologic symptoms after hyperbaric subarachnoid anesthesia with 5% lidocaine and 5% prilocaine. *Anesthesiology* 1998;**88**:624–8.

115 Axelrod EH, Alexander GD, Brown M, Schork MA. Procaine spinal anesthesia: a pilot study of the incidence of transient neurologic symptoms. *J Clin Anesth* 1998;**10**:404–9.

116 Bergeron L, Girard M, Drolet P, Grenier Y, Truong HHL, Boucher C. Spinal procaine with and without epinephrine and its relation to transient radicular irritation. *Can J Anaesth* 1999;**46**:846–9.

# 9: Complications of local and regional anaesthesia

JEAN-JACQUES ELEDJAM, JACQUES RIPART, ERIC VIEL

Regional anaesthesia (RA) brings many potential benefits for a wide variety of surgical procedures. It also has risks and potential complications which are frequently overemphasised and used as reasons to prefer general anaesthesia (GA). In fact, many complications are incidental and not due to the technique per se. Compared with GA, RA is frequently criticised for a purported higher complication rate. This assumption comes from two conceptual misunderstandings. First, there are still too many who consider that RA can be a good indication if GA is contraindicated or considered as high risk. This is a major misconception and one should remember that the anaesthetic risk is not modified by the choice of the technique, unless we consider peripheral nerve blocks. That is to say that potential risks are very often quite similar for a high-risk patient in both GA and spinal techniques. The second point is that, unlike GA, partial or total failure of RA is immediately apparent and immediately perceived by the patient, the anaesthetist, and the surgeon.

The risks and incidence of complications and litigation problems are very often overemphasised. Although the possible complications of RA are numerous and various, their incidence remains relatively low.[1-4] Broadly speaking, causes can be divided into complications due to the technique, complications due to anaesthetic drugs and solutions, and complications resulting from the patient's background and/or concurrent disease and related medications. Many complications are incidental and not due to the technique at all but some are the result of an incorrect or unsuitable technical approach and, consequently, are avoidable.[5]

## Complications of spinal anaesthesia

### Immediate complications

Inability to locate the subarachnoid space is rare, except in certain conditions such as in patients with major spinal deformations or ankylosing spondylitis. This should be detected during the anaesthetic consultation so that the technical approach can be adapted to the specific anatomical condition (e.g. puncture in sitting position instead of lateral decubitus, paramedian instead of median approach or any technique leading to an increased success rate).

Paraesthesia results from contact with a spinal nerve root and is resolved by withdrawing the needle a few millimetres. Recently, paraesthesiae have been shown to occur more frequently in patients with lumbar spine pathology.[6] Direct nerve trauma is exceptional and the occurrence of intense pain during puncture represents an absolute contraindication to injection of the anaesthetic solution and calls for immediate withdrawal of the needle. Failure to do so may result in intraneural injection responsible for nerve ischaemia, compression, and laceration, i.e. potential sources of severe sequelae.

Puncture of the dura mater with the introducer may result in a significant dural lesion followed by postdural puncture headache. Blood in the spinal needle is caused by puncture of a small vessel and the blood is rapidly flushed out by the cerebrospinal fluid (CSF). If the CSF does not clear, injection is contraindicated and the needle is withdrawn. The patient must be observed for symptoms of a possible spinal haematoma, and when indicated, treatment must be instituted as soon as possible.

## Complications of nerve blockade

### Cardiovascular effects

A prospective review of the cardiovascular side effects of spinal anaesthesia (SA) included hypotension (33%), bradycardia (13%), and dysrhythmias (2%).[7]

Hypotension is considered as a complication if the decrease in arterial blood pressure reaches 30% as compared to control values. It results from local anaesthetic-induced sympathetic blockade, which normally affects both the systemic resistance of arterial and capacitance systems. The decrease in systemic vascular resistance, together with venodilation and reduction of venous return, causes a decrease in arterial pressure, depending on the extent of sympathetic blockade and also of baroreflex responses in unblocked regions of the body. Usually, the arterial blood pressure decrease remains moderate if the upper dermatomal level of the neuraxial block is ≤T12 but it will be greater if it reaches T6, which would affect the splanchnic nerves and thereby increase splanchnic blood storage. SA may have deleterious haemodynamic consequences if the upper level of the block reaches T4, which will induce cardiac sympatholysis while the vagal tone remains unchanged. It results in negative chronotropic and inotropic effects leading to a reduction of cardiac output and to hypotension. The rapidity of the establishment of the block is also an important determining factor of haemodynamic response; titrated continuous spinal anaesthesia is better tolerated than single-shot spinal anaesthesia in terms of haemodynamics.

Effective prevention of hypotension is more effective than curative treatment. There are two clinically practical possibilities: vascular loading (crystalloids, dextrans, gelatins or hydroxyethyl starches) and intravenous sympathomimetic vasopressors (adrenaline, ephedrine, etilefrine, phenylephrine). In adult patients, it may be advisable to limit vascular loading to 500 ml (except in cases of predicted significant blood losses) in order to avoid urinary retention at the end of the procedure. In cardiac patients, it must also be avoided as excessive vascular loading may precipitate acute cardiac failure when the block wears off. Ephedrine (direct and indirect sympathomimetic, $\alpha$ and $\beta$-adrenergic agonist) is widely used, as is phenylephrine (mainly $\alpha$1-adrenergic agonist), in situations where excessive tachycardia must be prevented (i.e. coronary patients). Curative treatment of hypotension is also based on plasma expansion and vasoconstrictors.

## Nausea and vomiting

Arterial hypotension and/or excessive vagal tone (high sympathetic blockade) in spinal anaesthesia may result in nausea and vomiting. Prevention and treatment are based on administration of fluids and/or atropine intravenously. Otherwise, nausea and vomiting associated with spinal anaesthesia are quite rare, except when an opioid has been added to the local anaesthetic solution.

## Urinary retention

This is a relatively frequent problem of spinal anaesthesia (up to 40% in several series). Urinary retention results from sacral root blockade and can be precipitated by excessive fluid loading. Urinary bladder catheterisation may be required and repeated clinical examination for bladder distension should be consistently conducted during the whole postoperative period. In the setting of ambulatory surgery, natural voiding is often a mandatory criterion before allowing discharge of the patient after spinal anaesthesia.

## Backache

Back and lower back pain are thought to be caused by intervertebral ligament stretching resulting from relaxation of paravertebral muscles during spinal anaesthesia. This kind of back pain is distinctly different from the radiating transient neurological symptoms (TNSs) sometimes occurring after spinal anaesthesia (Chapter 8).

## Postdural puncture headache (PDPH)[3,8]

PDPH has long been considered a limitation of using spinal anaesthesia in young patients and parturients. Currently, thanks to a better understanding of its causes, PDPH in these categories of patients has become more of a complication of accidental dural puncture during epidural anaesthesia than following an intended dural puncture in spinal anaesthesia.[1,3,9]

PDPH is thought to result from CSF leakage through the puncture hole in the dura mater. The pressure difference between subarachnoid and epidural spaces ($+40$–$50$ cmH$_2$0 in the sitting position) then induces CSF leak, proportional to the size of the dural hole. When a patient with a decreased CSF volume and intrathecal pressure stands up, there is downward traction of neuraxial structures which are not damped by the fluid column. This results in stretching of meningeal envelopes and their vessels, which contain "stretch-sensitive receptors". PDPH may be amplified by local reflex vasodilatation, aimed at restoring the intracranial volume.

The incidence of PDPH is affected by several factors such as needle characteristics and the age of the patient.[3,10] Some 50 years ago, Dripps and Vandam[10] showed that the incidence of PDPH decreased with increasing age; for example, with the use of a 22 G Quincke bevel needle, the incidence was 10–20% in patients younger than 50 years, 5% at age 50–65 years, and 1–2% above 65 years.[10] The incidence of PDPH also increases with needle diameter.[10] Small-diameter needles are mandatory, especially in young adults and parturients, and 25–27 G needles undoubtedly represent the best compromise, as thinner diameter needles (e.g. 29 G) may be more difficult to use (needle bending, twisting, multiple punctures required).[11] The shape of the needle bevel is also important[12] and using pencil-point needles (Whitacre, Pajunk, Sprotte) instead of Quincke-type bevel needles dramatically reduces the incidence of PDPH. Other factors are also influential, such as the bevel of cutting-tip needles in relation to dural fibres. Although the anatomical basis is not clearcut, it has repeatedly been shown that insertion of the bevel parallel to the main direction of the elastic fibres reduces the size of the dural hole as compared to transverse insertion. The paramedian approach also results in a significant reduction of PDPH as compared to the median approach.[12,13] In the paramedian technique, and with the patient in the "curved" blocking position, the needle/dura angle will be smaller than in the midline technique and it is assumed that the more oblique puncture "channel" in the dura and arachnoid will be closed by the membranes.

The onset of PDPH takes place within 48 hours following anaesthesia, most often during the first hours. The intensity of headache increases with standing up or sitting and decreases in the horizontal position. Localisation is usually cervicooccipital, sometimes frontal or frontoorbital and sometimes with variable location over time. Other symptoms such as nausea,

138

vomiting, auditory (tinnitus, buzzing, hearing loss) and visual disorders (blurred vision, decreased visual acuity, phosphenes, diplopia) may also occur. Auditory disorders result from hypotension of the endolymph, while visual disorders result from stretching and/or compression of the cranial nerves, especially the sixth cranial nerve (abducens).

Many therapeutic approaches are found in the literature, schematically classified into three categories:[8] no treatment, measures of uncertain efficacy, and curative treatment. Most studies confirm that, within five days, significant numbers of PDPH disappear spontaneously or the intensity is markedly reduced. Such a natural history makes it understandable why so many different treatments have proved effective in the course of the first 5–7 days. Therefore, in many centres, the current consensus is not to treat before day 5. Nevertheless, any disabling PDPH with no spontaneous trend towards improvement after 48 hours may need definitive treatment.

Several treatments are of variable and debatable efficacy. Strict horizontal bedrest has only a symptomatic efficacy by decreasing the intensity of PDPH, but has neither preventive nor curative efficacy. By contrast, early ambulation seems to reduce the incidence of PDPH[14] by promoting inter-meningeal (arachnoid/dura) slip and non-alignment of the puncture path, thus decreasing CSF leak. Hyperhydration is not of special interest while normal hydration is essential in any case. PDPH is remarkably resistant to both opioid and non-opioid analgesics and multiple drug combinations may be inefficient and even hazardous. Intravenous caffeine may be useful in the early phase of PDPH as it induces meningeal vasoconstriction and appears effective in nearly 70% of cases.[15] In some centres, caffeine is in fact the first-line treatment of PDPH. Contraindications to caffeine treatment are epilepsy, toxaemia in pregnancy, and hypertension.

Definitive treatment of PDPH consists of an epidural injection of autologous blood, first described in 1960 as the epidural blood patch. This technically simple method is consistently effective in approximately 95% of cases.[16,17] Transient (24–48 hours) adverse effects have been reported, such as mild hyperthermia (38–38.5°) and low back pain. Its efficacy and the absence of severe adverse effects are such that it should be used whenever PDPH shows no trend towards spontaneous resolution. Often, complete resolution of headache is immediately obtained. The patient should be maintained in the decubitus position for 1–2 hours after the procedure. In case of failure, the blood patch may be repeated, usually with success, while some authors recommend an epidural infusion of normal saline.[18] Epidural blood patch does not preclude a future epidural anaesthesia.[19]

## Neurological complications

Although rare, neurological complications associated with spinal anaesthesia are nonetheless to be feared as they may give rise to devastating sequelae. Mechanisms are diverse but a direct relationship with spinal anaesthesia may often be difficult to establish.

### Ischaemia

Spinal cord ischaemia may result from excessive hypotension or local vasoconstriction. It generally gives rise to the anterior spinal artery syndrome comprising motor paraplegia with loss of thermoalgesic sensitivity and sphincter disorders. This is easily explained, considering that the posterior part of the spinal cord is vascularised by 4–6 arteries while blood supply to the anterior cord depends on a single artery (arteria radicularis anterior magna or Adamkievicz's artery). Nevertheless, a relationship with spinal anaesthesia per se has not been established with certainty as this syndrome has also developed following general anaesthesia.

Among other causes of spinal cord ischaemia, it has been suggested that exaggerated and prolonged hyperlordosis could in rare instances be responsible for a compromised venous circulation leading to spinal cord venous infarction.[20]

### Paraesthesia and neurological sequelae

Needle and catheter trauma rarely results in permanent neurological injury. Earlier large-scale follow-up studies on spinal anaesthesia[21,22] have not been able to show any clear relationship between the frequency of paraesthesia during needle placement and the frequency of persisting pain. More recently, the first reports of a more obvious relationship ("association") between spinal needle-elicited paraesthesia and long-term postanaesthetic paraesthesia[23] or between spinal needle-elicited paraesthesia and radiculopathy, cauda equina syndrome or paraplegia[24] have been published. However, the exact roles of the needle, catheter or local anaesthetic in the mechanism of the neurological damage remain speculative.

### Preexisting neurological disorders

Acute neurological disorders are rare but are reported, again with no clearcut relationship with the technique. Rare cases of neural dysfunction due to slow medullar compression, intracranial lesion, and even puncture of an angiomatous structure have been revealed after spinal or epidural anaesthesia. Such cases are exceptional and impossible to foresee or prevent. Nevertheless, any persistent headache and/or any persistent neurological deficit are indications for thorough diagnostic examinations. In spite of the fact that a definitive causal relationship has never been proven between the exacerbation of neurological symptoms and regional anaesthesia, some anaesthesiologists regard spinal anaesthesia as relatively or even absolutely contraindicated in patients with multiple sclerosis and herpes zoster infection.

*Infectious complications*

Infectious complications are exceptional unless there are serious faults in antisepsis, sterility or technique.[2] Recently, a case of postspinal anaesthesia meningitis was reported, with the same bacteria in the patient's CSF as in the anaesthetist's oropharynx.[25] Therefore, spinal and epidural anaesthesia should be performed under strict asepsis with the anaesthesiologist wearing surgical mask and gloves.

## Spinal complications of local anaesthetics[26]

Along with the development of spinal microcatheters and a renewed interest in continuous spinal anaesthesia techniques, several cases of cauda equina syndrome were reported, leading the US Food and Drug Administration (FDA) to withdraw microcatheters from the market in 1992.

The cauda equina syndrome includes symptoms like bladder and bowel dysfunction, variable perineal sensory deficit, and lower limb paresis, slowly progressing over several days or weeks. Diagnosis is based on clinical symptoms and confirmed by electromyography. This rare complication has been linked with continuous SA where doses of local anaesthetics greater than normal were administered.[27] It has become obvious that the neural damage is not directly related to the catheters but rather to maldistribution of high doses of local anaesthetics, resulting in high concentrations in immediate contact with sacral nerve roots. Recommendations have been proposed[28] regarding catheterisation and the type of local anaesthetic solution, including limitation of continuous spinal anaesthesia to individual patients in whom a strong benefit/risk ratio from this anaesthetic technique would be expected.

Transient neurologic symptoms (TNSs) have also been reported following single-shot spinal injections,[29,30] mainly with 5% lignocaine in hyperbaric solutions, with an incidence of 15%.[31] TNSs, earlier called transient radicular irritation (TRI), have also been reported with 2% lidocaine, 0.5% amethocaine (tetracaine), and 4% mepivacaine but rarely with 0.5% bupivacaine, the latter usually being considered the safest in terms of local neurotoxicity.[32] TNSs are a syndrome-like state comprising variable pain radiating to the buttocks and legs after recovery of the block with no objective neurological signs at clinical examination. Speculations about the mechanisms are presented in more detail in Chapter 8.

# Complications of epidural anaesthesia

## Immediate complications

*Anaesthetic failure and inadequacies*
Spinal deformaties may complicate the approach to the epidural space.[33]

Such patient-related aspects must be detected during the preoperative anaesthetic consultation, in order to adapt the technique (position of the patient, choice of needle, midline vs paramedian approach, etc.) to the specific characteristics.

Total failure of epidural anaesthesia (EA) and/or a patchy block is frequently blamed on anatomical abnormalities and/or defective anaesthetic solution. In fact, these are more often consequences of poor anaesthetic skill or inadequate technical choices; for example, a mistake in the choice of the injected volume or concentration of the local anaesthetic solution. Patchy anaesthesia may result from compartmentalisation of the epidural space due to epidural adherences (e.g. spina bifida occulta, history of laminectomy or chemonucleolysis). Incomplete anaesthesia can also be secondary to aberrant catheter paths. The rate of failure ranges from 2.4% if the local anaesthetic is injected through the needle to 12% if the local anaesthetic is injected through the catheter. The catheter path is indeed unpredictable, especially if it is inserted more than 5 cm. The catheter can exit through an intervertebral foramen, giving incomplete anaesthesia or even a peripheral nerve block. A wide range of clinical blocks is in fact possible from no anaesthesia to extensive nerve block. In rare cases, restricted or unilateral anaesthesia may result from existing connective membraneous barriers in the epidural space.[34]

The technique for location of the epidural space may also cause inadequate anaesthesia. The loss of resistance to air technique may cause formation of epidural air bubbles,[35] preventing uniform spread of the local anaesthetic solution and giving rise to a patchy distribution of anaesthesia.

*Bloody tap*

A bloody tap may occur when an epidural vein is punctured by the needle or by the epidural catheter, which occurs more often in obstetric than non-obstetric patients. If the bleeding is persistent, the needle or catheter should be withdrawn and the procedure repeated in an adjacent intervertebral space, if possible. Then, if there is no bleeding, the epidural local anaesthetic solution can be injected carefully and fractionated. Such a patient must be observed with special attention for possible symptoms of systemic intoxication and development of spinal haematoma.

*Paraesthesia*

Paraesthesia may result from contact of the needle with a nerve root and is resolved by withdrawing the needle a few millimetres. The incidence varies from 5% to 25%.[36] Auroy and co-workers[24] found that occasionally, transient radiculopathy and even paraplegia may follow epidural anaesthesia, whether paraesthesia during needle or catheter placement has occurred or not.

*Accidental dural puncture*

The incidence of a direct accidental puncture of the dura with a Tuohy needle ranges from 0.5% to 2%.[36] Secondary perforation of the dura by the epidural catheter is more rare. Consequences may be immediate or delayed. If a large volume of local anaesthetic is injected, the immediate complication may be total spinal anaesthesia. A rapidly spreading extensive blockade is responsible for cardiovascular collapse and apnoea. Symptomatic treatment includes ventilatory support (tracheal intubation, mechanical ventilation), vascular loading, and/or vasopressors. Provided treatment is immediate, uneventful recovery and favourable outcome can be achieved. A delayed consequence of accidental dural puncture with an epidural needle is PDPH, with an incidence of approximately 50%. The success rate of prophylactic injection of normal saline via the catheter (repeated boluses or continuous infusion) varies considerably. Due to an equivocal efficacy and an additional procedure-related risk, a prophylactic blood patch in accidental dural puncture is usually not recommended.[36]

Instead of injection into the subarachnoid space, injection in the subdural space, i.e. between dura mater and pia arachnoid, may also occur. Because of a lower compliance and a greater longitudinal distribution of the injected solution, a larger spread of the block will occur compared to expected epidural extension. The incidence varies from 0.1% to 0.8%,[36] increased incidence being related to previous back surgery. Symptoms are slowly progressive, sometimes mimicking incomplete or patchy epidural anaesthesia. Hypotension may be the first symptom. A subdural block is usually weak and patchy and resolves faster than epidural or spinal block. If any doubt exists, injection of contrast medium and radiographic examination will confirm the incorrect position of the catheter.

## Hypotension

In epidural anaesthesia, arterial hypotension is secondary to local anaesthetic-induced sympathetic blocks as previously described in association with spinal anaesthesia. It may develop a little slower but it requires similar therapeutic measures as in spinal anaesthesia. In some instances, clinical advantage has been gained from this predictable arterial hypotension and, occasionally, total hip replacement may be performed under controlled epidural hypotensive anaesthesia.[37]

Back pain and low back pain are frequent, especially in obstetrics.[36] Such symptoms usually result from relaxation of paravertebral muscles and are encouraged by arthrosis, obesity, and previous spine surgery. Multiple attempts with the needle may increase the incidence of back ache by causing direct trauma and haemorrhage into vertebral ligaments and periosteum.

## Neurological complications

The incidence of neurological complications, excluding PDPH, after epidural blocks has been reported to vary from 0.1/10 000 in a survey of only obstetric patients[38] to 1.8/10 000 in a mixed patient population,[39] probably secondary to direct needle or catheter trauma. Resulting muscular weakness and hypoaesthesia may last from several weeks to several months. When evaluating complications after anaesthesia, surgical factors such as patient position during and after surgery and the use of a tourniquet in lower extremity surgery should also be considered as possible aetiological factors. Back pain and low back pain in particular, after epidural analgesia or anaesthesia, are frequent sequelae in obstetric patients.[36]

### Infections

Meningitis has been rarely reported, in spite of the fact that epidural anaesthesia has been used in febrile patients, as well as in septic patients.[40]

The incidence of epidural abscesses related to epidural catheters is low,[41,42] a rough estimate being 15 abscesses per 1 million epidural anaesthesia procedures.[43] From the first report in 1974 until the beginning of the 1990s, 42 cases of epidural abscesses in connection with epidural anaesthesia and analgesia via catheters were published.[42] A spinal haematoma may predispose to the development of an epidural abscess.[43] Among other risk factors are epidural injection of steroids,[44] underlying sepsis, diabetes, and depressed immune status. Duration of epidural catheterisation does not appear as a decisive factor as symptoms of epidural abscess may appear between one and 60 days after catheter insertion.[45] An abscess may be associated with early back pain following epidural anaesthesia and/or localised tenderness and/or symptoms of spinal cord compression, along with infectious symptoms.

Prompt emergency imaging, using CT scan or preferably MRI, is necessary for establishing early diagnosis and treatment. Staphylococcus is the most common infectious microorganism and surgical treatment (decompressive laminectomy) is most often indicated combined with antibiotic therapy (for a minimum of 2–6 weeks).[46]

### Haematomas

Magnetic resonance imaging shows that epidural needles and catheters frequently cause vascular trauma associated with minimal haemorrhage, spontaneously resolving without any symptoms and/or sequelae. Sometimes multiple puncture attempts may cause trauma and haemorrhage in the intervertebral ligament and even the periosteum, causing back ache for several weeks.

Subarachnoid bleeding or epidural haematomas are reported with a low incidence, less than one in 150 000 epidural blocks.[47] This complication is

144

considered more rare than spontaneous spinal haematoma and therefore a cause-and-effect relationship is difficult to establish. The risk will increase with multiple and/or traumatic intervertebral puncture and/or needle or catheter placement difficulties and also in patients on anticoagulant or antithrombotic treatments.[48,49] Neuraxial anaesthesia (epidural and spinal) must therefore follow certain safety rules,[45,48] i.e. coagulopathy is a definite contraindication, while ongoing treatment with acetylsalicylic acid is considered a relative contraindication. In addition, low-molecular weight heparins (LMWH), heparin, and potent NSAIDs (e.g. ketorolac,[50] diclofenac) may increase the risk of bleeding and therefore combination with epidural and spinal anaesthetics is acceptable only if there is a clearcut reason to choose one of these techniques instead of general anaesthesia. The safety of combining neuraxial RA with LWMH has been documented in several hundred thousands of patients[37,39,51] but recommended dosages must be strictly respected, avoiding raising the doses to full therapeutic level.[51] In addition, attention must be paid to timing of thromboprophylaxis administration; that is, 10–12 hours before neuraxial regional anaesthesia. The same timing is recommended for epidural catheter removal.[3,52] On the other hand, the initial dose of the most recent thromboprophylactic agents, the thrombin antagonists, can be administered immediately after the induction of a central neuraxial block.

According to Bromage,[42] multiple factors such as direct trauma to nervous tissues, insufficient supervision and training of novice physicians, lack of manual dexterity, inattention, poor judgement, and ignorance may predispose to the development of neurological complications. In addition, teaching nursing personnel in charge of postoperative surveillance about the nature of early symptoms of spinal cord compression is a key point for the prevention of neurological catastrophes.[45] Monitoring of leg weakness as an early symptom of neurological complication and daily inspection of the skin at the catheter insertion site are therefore crucial for early diagnosis and treatment.

## Complications of peripheral nerve blocks

Two types of complications may occur: unexpected extension of the block to neighbouring neurological structures and direct peripheral nerve damage. Damage to neighbouring viscera and vessels may also occur in several techniques.

### Complications of brachial plexus blocks

Due to the general use of large volumes of potent local anaesthetics in brachial plexus blocks, mild systemic toxic reactions and even generalised convulsions are sometimes encountered. Most of the complications probably occur with the interscalene approach, because puncturing or catheterisation imprecision may easily result in vascular, pleural or neural lesions. In principle, thanks to the aid of a nerve stimulator and with careful needle manoeuvring, the brachial plexus blocks are technically relatively simple to perform.

*Central extension: subarachnoid, subdural, and epidural injection*[53–57]

Central neural blockade is a potential complication of any nerve block performed in the paravertebral region. It has been described following lumbar plexus, intercostal, and paravertebral blocks and after brachial plexus anaesthesia.

Subarachnoid injection results either from needle misplacement into the intervertebral foramen (inappropriately deep placement of the needle bevel), usually at the C6–7 level, exceptionally at T1–2, or from puncture of a dural cuff. These cuffs are extensions of dura mater along nerve roots, through the intervertebral foramen which ends in front of the transverse process of the corresponding vertebrae. The risk of total spinal anaesthesia is greater than that of subdural anaesthesia.[55–57] In the latter case, clinical symptoms are identical to those of spinal anaesthesia but usually described as more slowly progressive. Total spinal anaesthesia is a severe complication, with rapidly progressing symptoms. As the injection is performed at the cervical level, unconsciousness, cardiovascular collapse, and respiratory arrest may occur almost instantaneously. Severe symptoms may occur following administration of even small volumes of local anaesthetics.[53] Provided ventilatory control (tracheal intubation, mechanical ventilation) and haemodynamic support (vascular loading, vasopressive agents) are rapidly given, symptoms are usually short-lived and, in most cases, the patient recovers without sequelae. Extension of the spread of the local anaesthetic solution to the epidural space has also been reported following the interscalene approach to the brachial plexus, after either single-shot injection through the needle[53] or catheter insertion at the interscalene level.[56]

The incidence of the central extension of brachial plexus blockade varies according to the technique, i.e. it is more common following the interscalene approach than the supraclavicular techniques. The highest risk of intrathecal injection is probably linked to Winnie's classic approach,[58] at the C5–6 level. This is because the needle is introduced laterally, perpendicular to the skin, and directed parallel to the main axis of the intervertebral foraminal canal. Thus, even when a correct motor response to nerve stimulation is obtained, it is difficult to estimate accurately the position of the needle in relation to the intervertebral foramen. Furthermore, in spite of the subarachnoid placement of the needle, the aspiration test is often negative. A modified technique seems preferable, for example, by introducing the needle medially, caudally and posteriorly.

*Phrenic nerve paralysis*

The incidence of ipsilateral phrenic nerve blockade following interscalene[59-61] and supraclavicular[62] approaches of the brachial plexus ranges from 35% to 100%. Urmey *et al*,[60] using ultrasonography, reported a 100% incidence, leading to a 25% temporary reduction in pulmonary function in patients undergoing interscalene block anaesthesia.[63] The incidence of hemidiaphragmatic paralysis is independent of the local anaesthetic in use,[64] of its concentration, and of its volume.[63-65] In healthy subjects, unilateral phrenic paresis has no adverse consequences. On the other hand, this approach should be avoided in patients who cannot tolerate a reduction in their ventilatory function, such as subjects with moderate to severe COPD, as it may precipitate an acute respiratory failure. In such patients, axillary or brachial canal approaches are preferable. Phrenic nerve block, which is usually benign and self-limiting, has also been described following other supraclavicular approaches than the interscalene approach.

*Intraarterial injection*

Inadvertent puncture or catheterisation[66] of the vertebral artery has been described and is responsible for immediate unconsciousness, without convulsions, resulting from the neurotoxic effects of bupivacaine.

*Stellate ganglion block*

Cervical sympathetic plexus blockade, resulting in Horner's syndrome, is relatively frequent, ranging from 18–75% in the interscalene technique to 46% in the supraclavicular technique.[53,63] Clinical symptoms are myosis, ptosis, enophthalmos, ipsilateral hemifacial redness and anhidrosis, which are often associated with successful interscalene brachial plexus block. Hoarseness, due to sympathetic blockade-induced swelling of the laryngeal mucous membrane, may also occur. Patients must be informed of these benign and always reversible events before the interscalene brachial plexus block is performed.

*Recurrent nerve block*

Recurrent nerve block has been described following the interscalene approach to the right brachial plexus, resulting in vocal paralysis or hoarseness. Because of an increased risk of aspiration due to unilateral paralysis of the vocal cords, oral food intake must be delayed until recovery.

*Pneumothorax*

The incidence of pneumothorax, due to the close anatomical relationship of the brachial plexus with the parietal pleura, varies from 0.6% to 6.1%.[67] Initially, clinical symptoms are often not noticed and diagnosis is frequently delayed. As this complication is mainly seen following the classic supraclavicular approach, this technique cannot be recommended for ambulatory surgery. Pneumothorax has also been described following interscalene and infraclavicular approaches. Many alternatives to the classic interscalene and supraclavicular approaches have been proposed in an attempt to avoid pneumothorax. Recommendations for good clinical practice are to limit needle depth insertion to 30 mm, to avoid needle insertion in the caudal direction, and to use neurostimulation for nerve location.

*Vascular damage*

In the case of accidental arterial puncture, whatever the technique, compression for at least five minutes must be applied in order to avoid the development of a large haematoma and subsequent fibrosis and nerve compression.[68] Ischaemia and axillary artery thrombosis have been described as a rare complication[69] and compressive haematoma with radial nerve compression has also been recently reported.[70] In a French survey, arterial punctures during brachial plexus blocks, without consequences, were quite frequent (37%).[58]

## Complications of lower limb plexus blocks

Complications of posterior lumbar plexus blocks are rare. Subcapsular renal haematoma and psoas muscle haematoma in a patient receiving LMWH[71] have been described. Accidental subarachnoid injections are exceptional. Epidural injection may occur a little more frequently, ranging from 1% to 16%.[71] Anterior approaches to this plexus, as well as sciatic nerve blocks, have no specific complications, except rare cases of neuropathies (direct nerve trauma) or compressive haematomas.

## Peripheral nerve damage

Although rare,[3,72] peripheral neuropathies represent a severe complication and must remain a constant concern.[52,72,73] They can be avoided by always using careful and accurate location techniques. Symptoms vary from short-lasting paraesthesiae and transient and mild dysaesthesiae to severe pain and permanent paresis.[2,53] In most cases, outcome is good with full recovery within a few days or weeks. Peripheral nerve damage may result from direct nerve trauma by the needle or from intraneural injection of local anaesthetics.

*Intraneural injection of local anaesthetics*

High-concentration local anaesthetics are myotoxic and neurotoxic[74] and care must be taken to avoid any inadvertent intraneural injection. In fact, local neurotoxicity is usually not the primary cause of nerve lesions. In the experimental work by Selander *et al*,[75] intrafascicular injections of local anaesthetic and/or saline solutions were shown to cause blood/nerve barrier damage and axonal degeneration. Intrafascicular injections are responsible for ischaemic damages which will result from high pressure exceeding capillary pressure for 10–15 min.[76]

An intraneural injection can be avoided by using a nerve stimulation instead of paraesthesia technique for nerve location.[77] Light paraesthesia occurring during nerve location will usually cause no harm, while severe, sharp, and excruciating pain at the beginning of the injection suggests that intraneural pressure is rising. This is a signal to stop injection immediately and to withdraw the needle. For this reason, performing regional anaesthesia requires awake patients and, consequently, blocks should not be performed in adult patients under general anaesthesia or deep sedation. Intraneural injections of local anaesthetics, leading to nerve fascicle disruption, are rare. In a French retrospective epidemiologic study,[53] two cases were reported following the axillary approach to the brachial plexus for hand surgery: one total paralysis with hyperaesthesia and hyperalgesia in the median nerve territory, and one total paralysis of the ulnar nerve.

The role of injection needles in nerve trauma remains controversial. In the experimental study by Selander et al.,[75] classic sharp-bevelled needles were associated with a higher incidence of nerve fascicular damage as compared to blunt-bevelled needles. The authors therefore suggested that a 45°-bevelled needle should be recommended for clinical use. This was not confirmed by Rice and McMahon,[73] who investigated needle injury in rat sciatic nerves. Indeed, they showed that when accidental nerve penetration occurred nerve injuries seemed to be more frequent, more severe and of longer duration when caused by short-bevelled needles as opposed to long-bevelled needles. The lowest injury rate was in fact associated with long-bevelled needles inserted parallel to the nerve fibres. In contrast, Baranowski and Buist[78] reported that paraesthesiae occurred exclusively following the use of long-bevelled needles.

Recommendations to completely avoid "paraesthesia searching techniques" are perhaps exaggerated, as claims that these techniques are dangerous remain unproven. Nevertheless, whatever the type of needle in use, Moore's classic assertion "No paraesthesia, no anaesthesia" cannot be whole-heartedly supported as paraesthesia is the sign of a direct contact between the needle and the nerve fibre and consequently of a nerve insult. Paraesthesiae can be avoided by using nerve stimulation, which should favour a more recent assertion "No paraesthesia, no dysaesthesia".[79] No controlled studies have been conducted comparing paresthesia with non-paraesthesia techniques with short-bevelled needles but extrapolation is possible from several studies showing that persistent neuropathies are more likely to occur following paraesthesia techniques. Selander and co-workers,[75] comparing the paraesthesia with the transarterial technique in axillary blocks, found incidences of neural damage of 2.8% and 0.8%, respectively.

In conclusion, care must be exercised before establishing any causative relationship between postoperative (postanaesthesia + postsurgery) neuro-logical complications and regional anaesthesia. Many other predisposing factors must be examined such as improper positioning on the operating table, intraoperative nerve compression or stretching, prolonged tourniquet inflation, surgical trauma, tight cast or dressing, diabetes mellitus and, preoperative existing peripheral neuropathy.[2,53]

# Complications of concomitantly administered opioids or sedatives

## Epidural and spinal opioids

Opioids have been widely used for epidural and spinal anaesthesia and analgesia, either alone or in combination with a local anaesthetic, for about 20 years.

Respiratory depression is a rare but severe complication of spinal opioid therapy.[80] The incidence does not seem to be dependent on the dose or the type of opioid.[52,81] The incidence is higher following subarachnoid than epidural administration: 5.5% versus 0.33% according to a national survey in Sweden.[82] After epidural application, respiratory depression may occur early, due to absorption of the opioid into blood. It may also be delayed after cephalad migration of the opioid within the CSF. The risk of delayed depression is greater with a hydrophilic opioid such as morphine than with the more lipophilic opioids (fentanyl, sufentanil). This risk, although rare, justifies close clinical monitoring (respiratory rate, sedation) of patients receiving (or who have received) spinal opioids. Monitoring must be continued for at least 12 hours following injection or the end of continuous infusion. Treatment of respiratory depression is with intravenous naloxone and oxygenation. Tracheal intubation and mechanical ventilation may be necessary in cases of respiratory arrest and also if buprenorphine has been employed because the effects of this agonist-antagonist-type opioid are poorly reversed by naloxone.

The incidence of pruritus associated with spinal opioids seems to vary from study to study. In the study by Ballantyne and co-workers,[83] it was approximately 10% and after caesarean section an incidence of 40–58% was reported.[84] Urinary retention is more frequent in men than in women and its incidence ranges from 22% to 40%.[85,86] Nausea and vomiting after epidural morphine also seem to occur at a frequency of 20–40%.[84,86]

## Intravenous sedatives

Mild sedation is frequently used in combination with regional anaes-thesia to either facilitate technical performance of the block or improve the patient's comfort during surgery under regional anaesthesia. Agents used are most often benzodiazepines (midazolam) or propofol. In rare circumstances (e.g. when pain is involved) opioids (e.g. fentanyl) may also be used for sedation. The main risk of complementary sedation is respiratory depression and hypoxaemia, as all the agents used may potentiate the respiratory depressant effect of spinal techniques, in healthy volunteers as well as in elderly patients.[87–89]

Whichever agent is used, there is an absolute necessity for adequate monitoring and close supervision of such patients during surgery and in the immediate postoperative period. One must therefore emphasise the need to carefully consider the indications for sedation during regional anaesthesia and to ensure flawless safety of the patient. Guidelines include the maintenance of permanent verbal and visual contact with the patient throughout the procedure and monitoring of at least ECG, non-invasive blood pressure, and pulse oximetry.[89] In deeply sedated patients, the monitoring of $PCO_2$ in the exhaled air (sampling catheter tip in the nostril) helps with the verification of an open airway and spontaneous respiration.

1   Tanaka K, Watanabe R, Harada T, Tan K. Extensive application of epidural anesthesia and analgesia in a university hospital. Incidence of complications related to technique. *Reg Anesth* 1993;**18**:34–8.

2   Wedel DJ. Complications of regional and local anesthesia. *Curr Opin Anaesthesiol* 1993;**6**:830–4.

3   Eledjam J-J, Viel E, van Roy C. Les complications des anesthésies locorégionales. In: Coriat P, ed. *Les situations critiques au bloc opératoire*. Paris: Arnette, 1996:337–69.

4   Dahlgren N, Törnebrandt K. Neurological complications after anaesthesia. A follow-up of 18000 spinal and epidural anaesthetics performed over three years. *Acta Anaesthesiol Scand* 1995;**39**:872–80.

5   McDonald R. Problems with regional anaesthesia: hazards or negligence? *Br J Anaesth* 1994;**73**:64–8.

6   Tetzlaff JE, Dilger JA, Wu C, Smith MP, Bell G. Influence of lumbar spine pathology on the incidence of paresthesia during spinal anesthesia. *Reg Anesth Pain Med* 1998;**23**:560–3.

7   Carpenter RL, Caplan RA, Brown DL, Stephenson C, Wu R. Incidence and risk factors for side effects of spinal anesthesia. *Anesthesiology* 1992;**76**:906–16.

8   Viel E, Eledjam JJ. Les céphalées post-ponction lombaire. *Med Ther* 1996;**2**:143–9.

9   Giebler RM, Scherer RV, Peters J. Incidence of neurologic complications related to thoracic epidural catheterization. *Anesthesiology* 1997;**86**:55–63.

10  Dripps RD, Vandam LD. Long-term follow-up of patients who received 10098 spinal anesthetics. *JAMA* 1954;**156**:1486–92.

11  Dahl JB, Schultz P, Anker-Möller E. Spinal anaesthesia in young patients using a 29G needle: technical considerations and an evaluation of postoperative complaints compared with general anaesthesia. *Br J Anaesth* 1990;**64**:178–82.

12  Ready LB, Cuplin S, Haschke RH, Nessly M. Spinal determinants of transdural fluid leak. *Anesth Analg* 1989;**69**:457–60.

13  Hatfalvi BI. Postulated mechanisms for postdural puncture headache and review of laboratory model. Clinical experience. *Reg Anesth* 1995;**20**:329–36.
14  Cook PT, Davies MJ, Beavis RE. Bed rest and post-lumbar puncture headache. *Anaesthesia* 1989;**44**:389–91.
15  Baumgarten RK. Should caffeine become the first-line treatment for postdural puncture headache? *Anesth Analg* 1987;**66**:913–22.
16  DiGiovanni AJ, Galbert MW, Wahle WM. Epidural injection of autologous blood for postlumbar puncture headache. II: Additional clinical experiences and laboratory investigation. *Anesth Analg* 1972;**51**:226–32.
17  Seebacher J, Ribeiro V, Le Guillou JL *et al*. Epidural blood patch in the treatment of postdural puncture headache: a double blind study. *Headache* 1989;**29**:630–2.
18  Baysinger CL, Menk EJ, Harte E, Middaug HR. The successful treatment of dural puncture headache after failed epidural blood patch. *Anesth Analg* 1986;**65**:1242–4.
19  Hebl JR, Horlocker TT, Chantigian RC, Schroeder DR. Epidural anaesthesia and analgesia are not impaired after dural puncture with or without epidural blood patch. *Anesth Analg* 1999;**89**:390–4.
20  Skouen JS, Wainapel SF, Willock MM. Paraplegia following epidural anesthesia. A case report and literature review. *Acta Neurol Scand* 1985;**72**:437–43.
21  Vandam LD, Dripps RD. A long-term follow-up of 10098 spinal anesthetics. II. Incidence and analysis of minor sensory neurological defects. *Surgery* 1955;**38**:463-9.
22  Philips OC, Ebner H, Nelson AT, Black MH. Neurological complications following spinal anesthesia with lidocaine. A prospective review of 10440 cases. *Anesthesiology* 1969;**30**:284–9.
23  Horlocker TT, McGregor DG, Matsushige DK, Schroeder DR, Besse JA. A retrospective review of 4767 consecutive spinal anesthetics: central nervous system complications. *Anesth Analg* 1997;**84**:578–84.
24  Auroy Y, Narchi P, Messiah A, Litt L, Rouvier B, Samii K. Serious complications related to regional anesthesia: results of a prospective survey in France. *Anesthesiology* 1997;**87**:479–86.
25  Duflo F, Allaouchiche B, Mathon L, Chassard D. Bacterial meningitis following combined obstetric spinal and epidural anesthesia. *Ann Fr Anesth Reanim* 1998;**17**:1286.
26  Peyton PJ. Complications of continuous spinal anaesthesia. *Anaesth Intens Care* 1992;**20**:417–38.
27  Rigler ML, Drasner K, Krejcie TC *et al* Cauda equina syndrome after continuous spinal anesthesia. *Anesth Analg* 1991;**72**:275–81.
28  American Society of Regional Anesthesia. Consensus statement on guidelines for the safe use of continuous spinal anesthesia. ASRA News, Milwaukee, February 1994:2–3.
29  Pollock JE, Neal JM, Stephenson CA, Wiley CE. Prospective study of the incidence of transient radicular irritation in patients undergoing spinal anesthesia. Anesthesiology 1996;**84**:1361–7.
30  Freedman J, Li D, Drasner K *et al*. Risk factors for transient neurologic symptoms after spinal anesthesia: an epidemiologic study of 1863 patients. *Anesth Analg* 1998;**89**:633–41.
31  Malinowski JM, Pinaud M. Neurotoxicité médullaire des agents anesthésiques. In: Anesthésie Réanimation, Conférences d'Actualisation 1997, SFAR ed, Elsevier: Paris, 1997:211–19.

32  Hitler A, Rosenberg PH. Transient neurological symptoms after spinal anaesthesia with 4% mepivacaine and 0.5% bupivacaine. *Br J Anaesth* 1997;**79**:301–5.

33  Sprung J, Bourke DL, Grass J *et al.* Prediction of the difficult neuraxial block: a prospective study. *Anesth Analg* 1999;**89**:384–9.

34  Blomberg R. The dorsomedian connective tissue band in the lumbar epidural space of humans. *Anesth Analg* 1986;**65**:747–52.

35  Saberski LR, Kondamuri S, Osinubi OY. Identification of the epidural space: is loss of resistance to air a safe technique? A review of the complications related to the use of air. *Reg Anesth* 1997;**22**:3–14.

36  Datta SJ. Complications of regional analgesia and anaesthesia. In: van Zundert A, ed. *Highlights in pain therapy and regional anaesthesia, vol. VII.* Cyprus: Hadjigeorgiou, 1998:21–7.

37  Sharrock NE, Mineo R, Urquhart B. Haemodynamic effects and outcome analysis of hypotensive extradural anesthesia in controlled hypotensive patients undergoing total hip arthroplasty. *Br J Anaesth* 1991;**67**:17–25.

38  Scott DB, Hibbard BM. Serious non-fatal complications associated with extradural block in obstetric practice. *Br J Anaesth* 1990;**64**:537–41.

39  Kane RE. Neurologic deficits following epidural or spinal anesthesia. *Anesth Analg* 1981;**60**:150–1.

40  Jacobsen KB, Christiaensen MK, Carlsson P. Extradural anaesthesia for repeated surgical treatment in the presence of infection. *Br J Anaesth* 1995;**75**:536–40.

41  Ngan-Kee WD, Jones MR, Thomas P, Worth RJ. Extradural abscess complicating extradural anaesthesia for Cesarean section. *Br J Anaesth* 1992;**69**:647–52.

42  Bromage PR. Spinal extradural abscess: pursuit of vigilance. *Br J Anaesth* 1993;**70**:471–3.

43  Yuste M, Canet J, Garcia M, Gil MA, Vidal F. An epidural abscess due to resistant staphylococcus aureus following epidural catheterisation. *Anaesthesia* 1997;**52**:163–5.

44  Goucke CR, Graziotti P. Extradural abscess following local anaesthetic and steroid injection for chronic low back pain. *Br J Anaesth* 1990;**65**:427–9.

45  Breivik H. Neurological complications in association with spinal and epidural analgesia – again. *Acta Anaesthesiol Scand* 1998;**42**:609–13.

46  Horlocker TT, Wedel DJ. Regional anesthesia and infection. In: Finucane BT, ed. *Complications of regional anesthesia.* Philadelphia: Churchill-Livingstone, 1999:170–83.

47  Tryba M. Epidural regional anaesthesia and low molecular weight heparin: pro. *Anästh Intensivmed Notfallmed Schmerzther* 1993;**28**:179–81.

48  Horlocker TT, Heit JA. Low molecular weight heparin: biochemistry, pharmacology, perioperative prophylaxis and guidelines for regional anaesthetic management. *Anesth Analg* 1997;**85**:874–85.

49  Wulf H. Epidural anaesthesia and spinal haematoma. *Can J Anaesth* 1996;**43**:1260–71.

50  Thwaites BK, Nigus DB, Bouska GW, Mongan PD, Ayala EF, Merill GA. Intravenous ketorolac tromethamine worsens platelet function during knee arthroplasty under spinal anaesthesia. *Anesth Analg* 1996;**82**:1176–81.

51  Lumpkin MM. FDA public health advisory : reports of epidural or spinal hematomas with the concurrent use of low molecular weight heparin and spinal/ epidural anesthesia or spinal puncture. *Anesthesiology* 1998;**88**:27A–28A.

52 Viel E, Bruelle P, Eledjam J-J. Anesthésie péridurale et rachianesthésie chez l'adulte. In: Bonnet F, Eledjam J-J, eds. *Actualité en anesthésie locorégionale*. Paris: Arnette, 1995:81–132.

53 Eledjam J-J, Bruelle P, Lalourcey L, Viel E. Diagnosis and mechanisms of neurological complications after brachial plexus blocks. In: van Zundert A, ed. *Highlights in pain therapy and regional anaesthesia, vol. V*. Barcelona: Permanyer Publications, 1996:187–95.

54 Eledjam JJ, Viel E, Bruelle P. Gestion des complications des anesthésies locorégionales. In: Bonnet F, Eledjam J-J, eds. *L'anesthésie locorégionale*. Paris: Arnette-Blackwell, 1994:165–90.

55 Dutton RP, Eckhardt WF, Sunder N. Total spinal anesthesia after interscalene blockade of the brachial plexus. *Anesthesiology* 1994;**80**:939–41.

56 Cook LB. Unsuspected extradural catheterization in an interscalene block. *Br J Anaesth* 1991;**67**:473–5.

57 Tetzlaff JE, Yoon HJ, Dilger J, Brems J. Subdural anesthesia as a complication of an interscalene brachial plexus block. *Reg Anesth* 1994;**19**:357–9.

58 Dupré LJ. Blocs périphériques du membre supérieur chez l'adulte. In: Bonnet F, Eledjam J-J, eds. *Actualité en anesthésie locorégionale*. Paris: Arnette, 1995:165–87.

59 Pere PP, Rosenberg PH, Bjorkenheim PH, Linden H, Salorinne Y, Tuominen M. Effect of continuous interscalene brachial plexus block on the diaphragm motion and ventilatory function. *Acta Anaesthesiol Scand* 1992;**36**:53–7.

60 Urmey WF, Talts KH, Sharrock NE. One hundred percent incidence of hemidiaphragmatic paresis associated with interscalene brachial plexus anesthesia as diagnosed by ultrasonography. *Anesth Analg* 1991;**72**:498–503.

61 Urmey WF, McDonald M. Hemidiaphragmatic paresis during interscalene brachial plexus block: effects on pulmonary function and chest wall mechanics. *Anesth Analg* 1992;**74**:352–7.

62 Knoblanche GE. The incidence and aetiology of phrenic nerve blockade associated with supraclavicular brachial plexus block. *Anaesth Intens Care* 1979;**7**:346–9.

63 Urmey WF, Gloeger PJ. Pulmonary function changes during interscalene brachial plexus block: effects of decreasing local anesthetic injection volume. *Reg Anesth* 1993;**18**:244–9.

64 Casati A, Fanelli G, Cedrati V, Berti M, Aldegheri G, Torri G. Pulmonary function changes after interscalene brachial plexus anesthesia with 0.5% and 0.75% ropivacaine: a double-blinded comparison with 2% mepivacaine. *Anesth Analg* 1999;**98**:587–92.

65 Sala-Blanch X, Lazaro JR, Correa J, Gomez-Fernandez M. Phrenic nerve block caused by interscalene brachial plexus block: effect of digital pressure and a low volume of local anesthetic. *Reg Anesth Pain Med* 1999;**24**:231–5.

66 Tuominen MK, Pere P, Rosenberg PH. Unintentional arterial catheterization and bupivacaine toxicity associated with continuous interscalene brachial plexus block. *Anesthesiology* 1991;**75**:356–8.

67 Winnie AP. Plexus anesthesia. Vol. I. Perivascular techniques of brachial plexus block. Fribourg: Mediglobe SA, 1990:227–32.

68 Staal A, van Voorthuisen AE, Vandijk LM. Neurological complication following arterial catheterisation by the axillary approach. Br J Radiol 1966; 39: 115-16.

69 Ott B, Neuberger L, Frey HP. Obliteration of the axillary artery after axillary block. *Anaesthesia* 1989;**44**:773–4.

70  Ben David B, Stahl S. Axillary block complicated by hematoma and radial nerve injury. Reg Anesth Pain Med 1999;**24**:264–6.

71  Eyrolle L. Blocs du plexus lombaire. In: Bonnet F, Eledjam J-J, eds. *Nouvelles techniques en anesthésie locorégionale.* Paris: CRI, 1998:215–28.

72  Chambers WA. Peripheral nerve damage and regional anaesthesia. *Br J Anaesth* 1992;**69**:429–30.

73  Rice ASC, McMahon SB. Peripheral nerve injury caused by injection needles used in regional anaesthesia: influence of bevel configuration, studied in a rat model. *Br J Anaesth* 1992;**69**:433–8.

74  Lambert LA, Lambert DH, Strichartz GR. Irreversible conduction block in isolated nerve by high concentrations of local anesthetics. *Anesthesiology* 1994;**80**:1082–93.

75  Selander D, Dhuner KG, Lundborg G. Peripheral nerve injury due to injection needles for regional anaesthesia. An experimental study of acute effects of needle point trauma. *Acta Anaesthesiol Scand* 1977;**21**:182–8.

76  Selander D, Sjöstrand J. Longitudinal spread of intraneurally injected local anaesthetics. An experimental study of the initial distribution following intra-neural injections. *Acta Anaesthesiol Scand* 1978;**22**:622–34.

77  Selander D, Edshage S, Wolff T. Paresthesiae or not paresthesiae? *Acta Anaesthesiol Scand* 1979;**23**:27–33.

78  Baranowski AP, Buist RJ. Peripheral nerve damage and regional anaesthesia. *Br J Anaesth* 1993;**70**:593.

79  Gentili ME, Wargnier JP. Peripheral nerve damage and regional anaesthesia. *Br J Anaesth* 1993;**70**:594.

80  Ready LB, Loper KA, Nessly M, Wild L. Postoperative epidural morphine is safe in surgical wards. *Anesthesiology* 1991;**75**:452–6.

81   Etches RC, Sandler AN, Daley MD. Respiratory depression and spinal opioids. *Can J Anaesth* 1989;**36**:165–85.

82  Gustafsson LL, Schildt BB, Jacobsen K. Adverse effects of extradural and intrathecal opiates: report of a nationwide survey in Sweden. *Br J Anaesth* 1982;**54**:479–86.

83  Ballantyne JC, Loach AB, Carr DB. Itching after epidural and spinal opiates. *Pain* 1988;**33**:149–60.

84  Fuller JG, McMorland JH, Douglas MJ, Palmer L. Epidural morphine for analgesia after cesarean section: a report of 4880 patients. *Can J Anaesth* 1990;**37**:636–40.

85  Lanz E, Theiss D, Riess W, Sommer U. Epidural morphine for postoperative analgesia: a double-blind study. *Anesth Analg* 1982;**61**:23–4.

86  Writer WDR, Hurtig JB, Edelist G et al. Epidural morphine prophylaxis of post-operative pain: report of a double-blind multicentre study. *Can Anaesth Soc J* 1985;**32**:330–8.

87  Munoz HR, Dagnino JA, Rufs JA, Bugedo GS. Benzodiazepine premedication causes hypoxemia during spinal anesthesia in geriatric patients. *Reg Anesth* 1992;**17**:139–42.

88  Gauthier RA, Dyck B, Chung F, Romanelli J, Chapman KR. Respiratory inter-action after spinal anesthesia and sedation with midazolam. *Anesthesiology* 1992;**77**:909–14.

89  Eledjam J-J, Bruelle P, Lalourcey L, Viel E. Sedation and regional anaesthesia. In: van Zundert A, ed. *Highlights in regional anaesthesia and pain therapy, vol. IV.* Barcelona: Permanyer Publications, 1995:136–44.

# Index

Note: page numbers in *italics* refer to figures and tables